CHILDHOOD CANCER

Information for the Patient and Family

SECOND EDITION

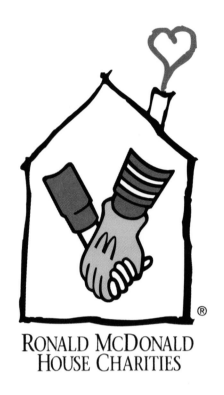

**RONALD MCDONALD
HOUSE CHARITIES**

Ronald McDonald House Charities provide comfort and care to children and families through their network of local Chapters currently serving in 32 countries. ■ The Charities make grants to non-profit organizations, primarily for programs that provide services aimed at improving the health and wellness of children, and provide support to Ronald McDonald Houses worldwide. ■ Their grant of US $281,437.00 to Children's Hospital of Hamilton Health Sciences Corporation underwrote the printing costs of two cancer resource guides. ■ These will be used to educate the 50,000 families of children who are newly diagnosed with cancer in North America over the next five years.

CHILDHOOD CANCER

Information for the Patient and Family

SECOND EDITION

Ronald D. Barr, MB, ChB, MD
Chief of Service, Hematology-Oncology
Children's Hospital
Hamilton Health Sciences Corporation
Professor of Pediatrics, Pathology and Medicine
McMaster University
Hamilton, Ontario
Canada

Mary Crockett
Susan Dawson, RN
Marilyn Eves, RN
Anthony Whitton, MB, BS
John Wiernikowski, PharmD

2001

BC Decker Inc

Hamilton • London

BC Decker Inc
20 Hughson Street South
P.O. Box 620, L.C.D. 1
Hamilton, Ontario L8N 3K7
Tel: 905-522-7017; 1-800-568-7281
Fax: 905-522-7839
E-mail: info@bcdecker.com
Website: www.bcdecker.com

Notice: The authors and publisher have made every effort to ensure that the patient care recommended herein, including choice of drugs and drug dosages, is in accord with the accepted standard and practice at the time of publication. However, since research and regulation constantly change clinical standards, the reader is urged to check the product information sheet included in the package of each drug, which includes recommended doses, warnings, and contraindications. This is particularly important with new or infrequently used drugs.

00 01 / CAD / 9 8 7 6 5 4 3 2 1

ISBN 1–55009–145–X
Printed in the United States

Sales and Distribution

United States
BC Decker Inc
P.O. Box 785
Lewiston, NY 14092-0785
Tel: 905-522-7017; 1-800-568-7281
Fax: 905-522-7839
E-mail: info@bcdecker.com
Website: www.bcdecker.com

Canada
BC Decker Inc
20 Hughson Street South
P.O. Box 620, L.C.D. 1
Hamilton, Ontario L8N 3K7
Tel: 905-522-7017; 1-800-568-7281
Fax: 905-522-7839
E-mail: info@bcdecker.com
Website: www.bcdecker.com

Foreign Rights
John Scott & Company
International Publishers' Agency
P.O. Box 878
Kimberton, PA 19442
Tel: 610-827-1640; Fax: 610-827-1671

U.K., Europe, Scandinavia, Middle East
Harcourt Publishers Limited
Customer Service Department
Foots Cray High Street
Sidcup, Kent
DA14 5HP, UK
Tel: 44 (0) 208 308 5760
Fax: 44 (0) 181 308 5702
E-mail: cservice@harcourt_brace.com

Australia, New Zealand
Harcourt Australia Pry. Limited
Customer Service Department
STM Division
Locked Bag 16
St. Peters, New South Wales, 2044
Australia
Tel: (02) 9517-8999
Fax: (02) 9517-2249
E-mail: stmp@harcourt.com.au
Website: www.harcourt.com.au

Japan
Igaku-Shoin Ltd.
Foreign Publications Department
3-24-17 Hongo
Bunkyo-ku,Tokyo, Japan 113-8719
Tel: 3 3817 5680
Fax: 3 3815 6776
E-mail: fd@igaku.shoin.co.jp

Singapore, Malaysia, Thailand, Philippines, Indonesia, Vietnam, Pacific Rim, Korea
Harcourt Asia Pte Limited
583 Orchard Road
#09/01, Forum
Singapore 238884
Tel: 65-737-3593
Fax: 65-753-2145

CONTRIBUTORS

Ronald D. Barr, Chief of Service, Pediatric Hematology-Oncology,
Professor of Pediatrics, Pathology and Medicine
Barb Cantwell, Nutritionist
Trish Case, Occupational Therapist
Stephen Couban, Fellow in Transfusion Medicine
Lynda Cranston, Professional Writer/Editor
Mary Crockett, Clinic Secretary
Susan Dawson, Pediatric Nurse (Oncology)
Marilyn Eves, Pediatric Nurse (Oncology)
John and Joanne Fabrizio, Parents
Laura Findlay, Cancer Patient
Dan Fleming, Chief Medical Director, North American Life Assurance Company
Steve and Wendy Gibbons, Parents
Jackie Halton, Pediatric Oncologist, Assistant Professor of Pediatrics
Nancy Heddle, Diagnostic Unit Manager, Assistant Professor of Pathology
Janet Jamieson, Pediatric Nurse (Oncology)
Mark Lane, Cancer Patient
Chantal Leblanc, Child Life Specialist
Brenden Mahon, Cancer Patient
Patti Massicotte, Fellow in Pediatric Thrombophilia
Mary Nolan, Professional Editor
Mohan Pai, Pediatric Oncologist, Professor of Pediatrics
Peter Pannozzo, Dental Consultant
John and Julia Parker, Parents
Ross Pennie, Pediatric Infectious Disease Specialist,
Associate Professor of Pathology and Pediatrics
Maria Restivo, Child Life Specialist
Marilyn Rothney, Pediatric Nurse (Oncology)
Toni Simpson, Pediatric Radiotherapy Liaison Nurse
Paula Smith, Cancer Patient
The Cancer Information Service
Victoria Tirone, Cancer Patient
Mark Walton, Pediatric Surgeon, Assistant Professor of Surgery and Pediatrics
Linda Waterhouse, Pediatric Oncology Social Worker
John Watts, Neonatologist/Ethicist, Professor of Pediatrics
Anthony Whitton, Pediatric Radiation Oncologist, Associate
Professor of Medicine and Pediatrics
John Wiernikowski, Clinical Pharmacist (Pediatric Oncology)
**Hematology-Oncology Service, Children's Hospital, Hamilton Health Sciences
Corporation and Division of Hematology-Oncology, Department of Pediatrics,
Faculty of Health Sciences, McMaster University**

FOREWORD

THE DRAMATIC IMPROVEMENTS IN THE OUTCOME OF CHILDHOOD CANCER WITH CONTEMPORARY TREATMENT HAVE NOT LESSENED THE ENORMITY OF THE IMPACT OF SUCH A DIAGNOSIS ON THE CHILD, PARENTS, AND SIBLINGS.

While the likelihood of cure has edged steadily upward, the road to cure remains a consummate challenge. ■ Travelling and transcending that road is aided by a comprehensive multidisciplinary team possessed of expertise and compassion and versed in the innumerable dimensions of holistic care. ■ To parents and families, concise, comprehensible, and transparent information about their child's illness, treatment and its complications, and the possible pitfalls, biologic and behavioral, on the road to recovery, cure, and reintegration into normal society is a weapon of enormous potency. ■ For it is this information and cumulative experience that arms them to face what they must in the struggle for a successful outcome.

The experienced staff of the Hematology-Oncology Service in the Children's Hospital of the Hamilton Health Sciences Corporation have done a remarkable job of assembling complex information about a complex disease process and its impact on child and family and conveying it coherently, succinctly, and compassionately. ■ The clarity of information makes this volume of value to parents and families in similar situations in other medical centers. ■ The diversity of authorship and breadth of understanding displayed speaks eloquently to the recognition that childhood cancer is more than a disease of cells or genes; it is a wrenching challenge to families and children. ■ A book such as this will facilitate communication between professionals and families and should prove an invaluable adjunct to coping with the challenge ahead.

Mark L. Greenberg
President, Canadian Society of Pediatric Hematology/Oncology
Continental President (North America)
International Society of Pediatric Oncology (SIOP)

PREFACE
SECOND EDITION

The IMPORTANCE OF CANCER IN CHILDREN, TO OUR SOCIETY AT LARGE, IS WELL ILLUSTRATED BY THE FACT THAT, EVEN THOUGH CANCERS IN CHILDREN REPRESENT ONLY 1 TO 2 PERCENT OF ALL CANCERS IN THE DEVELOPED WORLD, THESE DISEASES TOGETHER ARE THIRD MOST IMPORTANT IN TERMS OF POTENTIAL YEARS OF LIFE AFFECTED (AFTER BREAST AND LUNG CANCER) AND SECOND MOST IMPORTANT IN TERMS OF POTENTIAL YEARS OF LIFE SAVED (AFTER BREAST CANCER).

This reflects the life expectancy of healthy children and the high proportion of cases of cancer in childhood that are cured (almost 3/4 overall). ■ The relatively high cure rate is a direct consequence of the long-standing practice of entering children with cancer into randomized clinical trials that compare the best available therapy at the time with a new therapeutic strategy aimed at improving the prospects for survival, limiting the side effects of treatment or both.

Continuing improvement in survival rates for children with cancer often comes as a consequence of intensification of treatment. In turn, this poses the prospect of increased toxicity, which demands that more attention be paid to supportive care and prevention of side effects. ■ Examples of our ability to meet these demands successfully include the use of ondansetron (and similar drugs) and the administration of agents designed to stimulate the bone marrow (an ever-increasing family of compounds such as G-CSF).

Among the matters of particular relevance to the families of children with malignant diseases is the need to establish a formal network to provide concerted long-term follow-up for survivors of cancer in early life. ■ It is becoming ever more evident that such individuals can face major challenges beyond the cure of their original disease, and the spectrum of such potential disturbances to a return to an otherwise healthy life demands the attention of a wide array of health care professionals.

Looking to the future, we may anticipate further major advances ranging from the increasing empowerment of consumers of health care to continuing "miracles" of molecular biology, which will lead to a better understanding of cancer, open up the possibility of screening for these diseases (as well as the detection of "minimal residual disease"), provide an array of new substances to attack the malignant cell, and even enable clinicians to "turn off" the progression of malignancy (using gene therapy).

The purpose of this book is to provide a source of information and guidance for children with cancer and for their families. ■ It is intended to help them understand their new experiences and so reduce the fear that accompanies uncertainty. ■ The material is meant to complement and not substitute the essential continuing dialogue between families and members of the health care team. ■ The very use of this book should provoke and facilitate such discussions. ■ In addition, we hope that it will be utilized as a ready reference by families and as a resource for health professionals who are unfamiliar with the area of pediatric oncology.

The large number of individuals who have been involved in the development of this manual reflects the scope of expertise that is brought to bear on the management of children with malignant disease. ■ The format of the book is designed for ease of use, ready updating, flexibility between locations, and personalization. ■ Structurally, the layout will serve as a roadmap, taking the child and his family from diagnosis through treatment to ultimate outcome, which more and more often is that of cure. ■ There is a core of factual information that is suitable for all readers. ■ In addition, we encourage users to provide items of local information that are pertinent to a single hospital.

In the process of writing this book, we have involved patients, their families, and clinic staff, with the added support of professional editing. ■ We believe that the ultimate product is all the better for the variety of people who have contributed to its content.

The text has been written in a way that makes it user-friendly. ■ It is easily readable, with short summaries of many chapters aimed especially at the families of newly diagnosed children. ■ The inclusion of numerous illustrations highlights many of the important issues. ■ As is common practice, the child is referred to as "he" throughout, for the sake of simplicity and to avoid the clumsiness of using the combination of "he/she."

Although not all of the information contained in this book will be relevant to all children (for example, the brief description of so many different diseases), it will provide individual families with insight into the challenges faced by others, so encouraging the mutual support that plays such a crucial role in coping with cancer in childhood. ■ We trust that you will find this book to be of value and look forward to having your continuing input to future editions.

Ronald D. Barr, MB, ChB, MD
Professor of Pediatrics, Pathology and Medicine
McMaster University, Hamilton, Ontario
December 2000

ACKNOWLEDGMENTS

The editors wish to acknowledge Cure and Care for Children's Cancer and Leukemia, Help a Child Smile, several Rotary Clubs, and many individuals whose financial support enabled us to meet the development costs of this project.

We acknowledge the skill, forebearance, and encouragement of our publisher BC Decker Inc, in particular, the advice received from Rochelle and Brian Decker. ■ Special thanks are due to Herman Tauchert, whose imagination, expertise, and tireless effort contributed immeasurably to the "user-friendliness" of this book.

Of course we are indebted to the many contributors for their thoughtful input, and to Ronald McDonald Children's Charities, for without their investment our hopes may not have been realized. ■ The book is a "work in progress," as the care of children with cancer continues to evolve. ■ We invite our readers to send us their suggestions for improvement so that the next edition may even better meet their needs.

Hermann D. Tauchert

Mr. Tauchert is a graphic artist, designer and film animator, as well as a film producer and director. ■ He has more than 150 films to his credit, from educational and corporate films, to feature films that have premiered at Grauman's Chinese theater and at Radio City Music Hall. ■ Many of his films have received top honors worldwide. ■ Among these are the New York International and Atlanta Gold medals, and ten CINE Golden Eagle Awards. ■ His films have also earned the Silver Medal of Venice, Italy, and additional awards from Scotland, the Czech Republic, Australia, and Canada. ■ He has also received awards from Chicago, Houston and Columbus Film Festivals, which, among others, awarded him the Benjamin Franklin Award.

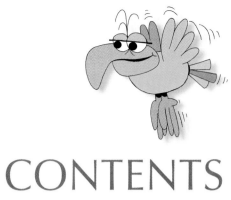

CONTENTS

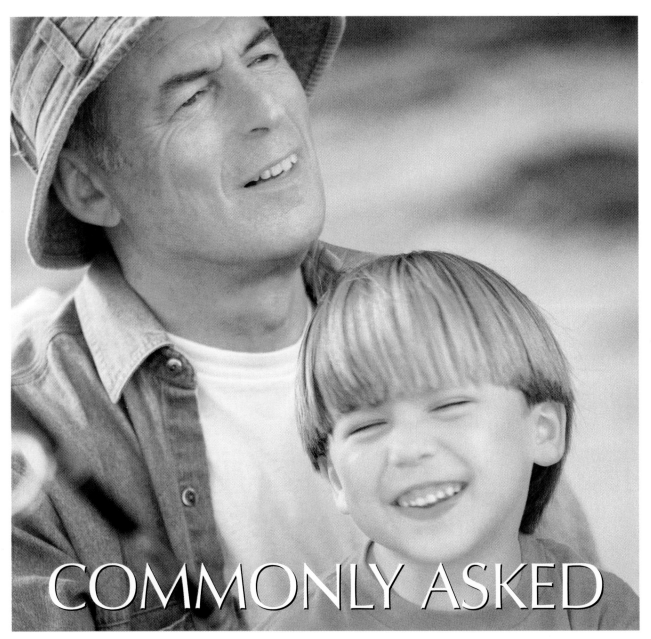

COMMONLY ASKED

QUESTIONS

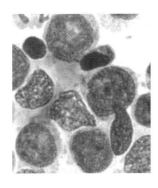

1. What is cancer?

Cancer is a group of diseases in which cells grow in an abnormal, uncontrolled way. ■ The body usually controls cell growth and development into mature cells. But, in cancer, this process is absent or doesn't work properly; as a result, cancer cells increase in number and spread. ■ We don't fully understand why normal cells mature and cancerous cells don't.

2 Why did my child get cancer?
In most instances, we don't know the answer to this question.

3. Where did the cancer come from?
Some parents are worried that a type of food or a poor appetite may have caused the cancer. ■ There is no proof that particular foods or eating habits cause childhood cancer. ■ Parents often wonder if something during pregnancy caused the cancer. ■ Except for abdominal x-rays (which are now uncommon during pregnancy), common events during pregnancy are not thought to cause childhood cancers. ■ Parents also ask if certain chemicals in the environment can cause cancer. There are many carcinogens (cancer-causing chemicals) in the environment, but, in almost all cases, there is no proof they cause cancer in children. ■ As well, x-rays for common things like broken bones and dental examinations do not increase a child's chances of developing cancer. ■ Finally, while we hear more and more about stress and illness, we don't know of any link between stress and the development of cancer in children.

4. Is it serious? Is there something you can do? Will my child die?
Without treatment, almost all cancers will progress and cause death. ■ Most cancers respond to treatment, and, while there are no guarantees, most children will survive their disease.

5. Will my child be cured?
There have been many advances in treating childhood cancer, and most children are being cured. ■ The chance for cure depends on the type and extent of the cancer when it is diagnosed. ■ Cure in childhood cancer means that the risk of the original disease returning is no greater than the risk faced by all healthy children of developing the same disease.

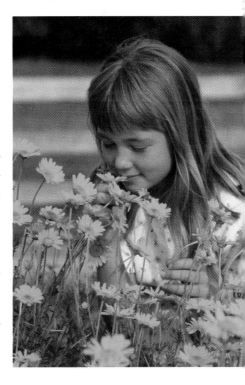

6. Would it have made a difference if we had come earlier? Is there something we should have noticed?
If some cancers are caught early, cure may be more likely. ■ But, in most cases, coming earlier to see the doctor doesn't have a large effect on the chance for cure. ■ It's often hard to tell early cancer symptoms apart from those of more common illnesses.

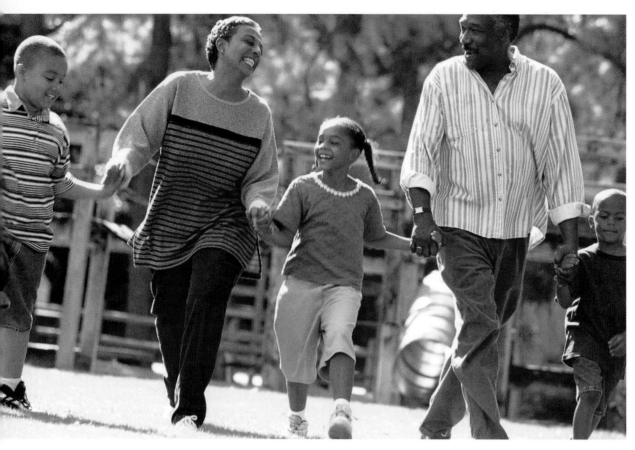

7. Will my other children get cancer? Cancer doesn't spread like the flu, so your other children, family, and friends can't catch cancer from your child. ■ The chances of other children in the same family developing the most common childhood cancers is the same as, or slightly more than, the general population. ■ In certain situations, this risk is increased, such as uncommon tumors that are inherited, the identical twin of a child with cancer, or perhaps families that are more likely to develop cancer.

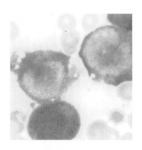

8. Will my child's cancer come back? Is he prone to another type of cancer? It is possible that the original disease may return (relapse), but the longer the remission (no symptoms or signs are present), the less likely a relapse will happen. ■ However, some forms of cancer and their treatment (such as radiation and chemotherapy) may cause other types of cancer to develop later.

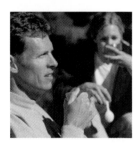

9. What should we do as parents? As parents, try to keep your family life as normal as possible, and try not to let your child's illness rule it completely. ■ This might take a lot of work and energy, but your child will be comforted and reassured.

10. Whom should we tell about this? What should we tell? Cancer is not something to be embarrassed about. ■ The more people know about your child's condition, the more they can help, support, and understand you. ■ Try to be open with family members and friends to avoid confusion. ■ Your child's siblings and your family need to be told as soon as possible. ■ The amount of information you give will depend on how much you know and how much your child understands. ■ Share information on a regular basis. ■ If your child is in school, it's important to tell the school about his condition. ■ If he needs to miss school during treatment, your child's nurse can help make it easier to go back once he is ready.

11. Will my child grow up normally? Survivors of childhood cancer usually grow up and develop normally. Growth and development may be delayed during the treatment period, but this is usually followed by a catch-up time. ■ Once treatment is finished, your child's growth will usually continue normally. Some parts of treatment may interrupt his growth (see Chapter 7 for more details). ■ Talk to the clinic staff if this is the case for your child. ■ During treatment, encourage your child to live a normal life. ■ Sometimes, he might not be able to take part in his usual activities. ■ But, otherwise, the answer is usually "yes" to the following questions: Can my child play with his friends, go to school, join clubs (e.g., Cubs, Brownies), attend camp and go on holidays, be involved in competitive sports, date, drive a car, take a job, and have a career? ■ Help your child to live life to its fullest and don't let cancer stand in his way!

12. Will treatment cause my child to be sterile? It depends on which treatment your child receives. Some treatments may cause sterility, but not everyone who is treated becomes sterile. ■ Remember, treatment may cause sterility, but it doesn't prevent normal sexual development.

13. Where can I find more information about my child's illness? Your clinic nurse can give you some information about your child's disease when he is first diagnosed. Plenty of other information is available too. ■ A health science library is one place you might go. Information there can be technical, but the staff can usually help you find what you need. There may be a library at your local Cancer Center, and your public library may be useful too. ■ Computer Oncolink, a text and multimedia service, is available through the Internet. ■ OncoLink can be accessed on the Internet using either the World Wide Web (http://cancer.med.upenn.edu/) or gopher (cancer.med.upenn.edu). ■ Always ask your child's health care team to look at any information you obtain to ensure that it is accurate and up to date.

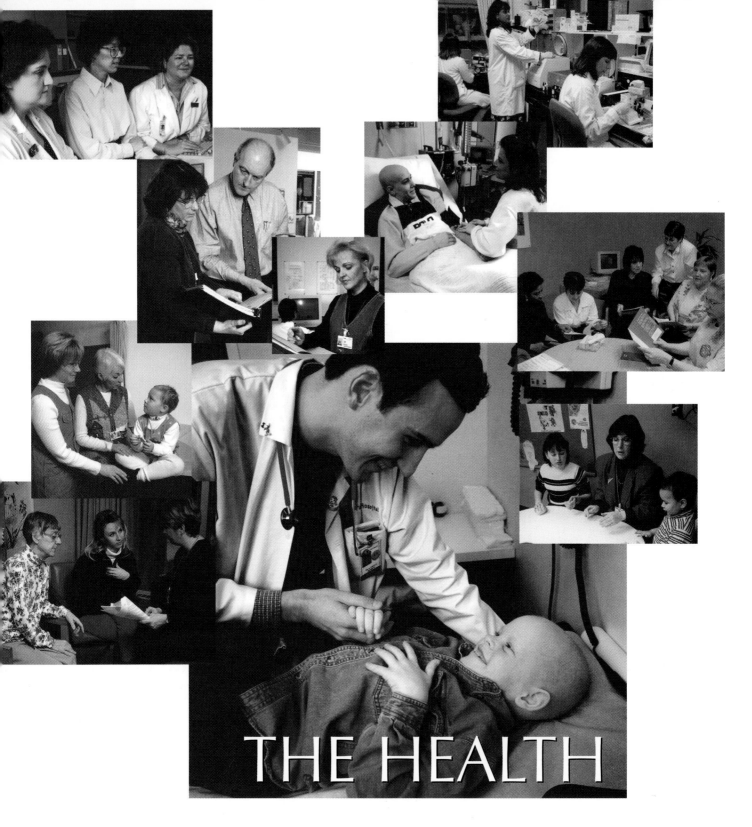

THE HEALTH
CARE TEAM

Clinic Doctors: When a child is thought to have cancer, he is sent to physicians who are trained to diagnose and treat children with cancer. ■ These physicians include pediatric oncologists (mainly responsible for the care of children with cancer), pediatric surgeons, and radiation oncologists.

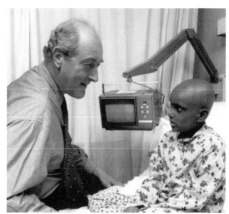

At the time of diagnosis, a pediatric oncologist will discuss with you the type and extent of cancer your child has, the forms of treatment available, possible complications and their management, and the long-term outlook. ■ Any new problem that comes up will also be discussed openly and fully with you. ■ Sometimes, other physicians who care for children with specific problems (e.g., lung, kidney, or heart disease) may be involved.

Some hospitals and all university medical centers serve also as teaching institutions, so physicians in training may be involved in your child's care. ■ These will include students (years one to four of medical school), interns (qualified physicians in their first or second year of post-graduate clinical training), residents (qualified physicians who are taking special training, usually in pediatrics), and fellows (fully trained specialists who are pursuing additional training in hematology/oncology).

Remember that the responsibility for your child's care is with the pediatric oncologist, who is on call at all times and may be reached through the hospital's paging system.

Clinic Nurses: Nurses who work in pediatric oncology outpatient clinics have special training in caring for families of children with cancer. ■ One nurse may be mainly responsible for you and your child. ■ She will be introduced to you at the time of diagnosis and will be your guide and main contact with the staff throughout the treatment program (including hospitalization) and beyond. ■ The nurse may be available through the hospital's paging system.

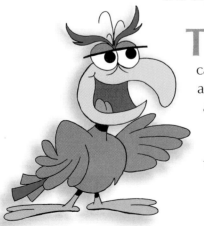

The nurse is a familiar face during a time when you and your child meet many new people and are trying to adjust to the diagnosis of cancer. ■ She will meet with you often to help you adjust and to answer your questions. ■ The nurse will educate you and your child about cancer, its treatment, and the effects on your child's lifestyle, both now and in the future. ■ The nurse encourages you to feel part of the team treating the disease and to expect that all examinations, tests, and treatments will be explained fully.

When your child is ready to leave the hospital, the nurse works with your family in planning his return home. ■ The goal is to achieve as normal a lifestyle as possible. ■ The discharge plans include co-ordinating your child's treatment program and visits to the clinic, his return to school, and your return to work. ■ Your nurse will contact the (American or Canadian) Cancer Society for help with transportation to and from the hospital, if this is necessary. ■ She will also introduce you and your child to other children with cancer and their families and to the support groups for parents and children.

Child Life Staff: The child life staff are trained to understand each stage of a child's development. ■ Their responsibility is to protect and improve the emotional well-being of each child in the hospital. ■ The child life staff explain to your child, in simple terms, all about the tests and treatments he will have and provide emotional support before and during these tests and treatments. ■ The child life staff help your child to co-operate and come to terms with his illness and its treatment.

Children and adolescents respond in many different ways to their illnesses and their treatment. ■ The child life staff will help you and your family understand and cope with these responses. ■ Play activity areas in inpatient and outpatient units are available for children and adolescents with cancer, as well as for their brothers and sisters. ■ Under supervision, expressing feelings and just having fun are encouraged there.

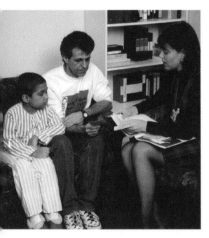

Social Worker: When children are affected by cancer, both they and their families experience stress, fear, and anxiety. ■ The social worker is there to help you cope with your problems and to help your family function in the healthiest way possible. ■ Some of the problems will relate to concerns for your child. ■ Others may have existed before your child's illness, and some may be a result of the changes that have happened in your family since the diagnosis of cancer. ■ You may wonder how to be strong when you're so frightened. ■ Financial problems or social isolation may, at times, seem too much to handle. Don't hesitate to take advantage of the special help offered to you, your child, and your entire family by the social worker.

Nutritionist: Along with you and the medical team, the nutritionist keeps a close eye on the nutritional status of your child and works to prevent your child from losing too much weight during treatment. ■ If your child stays well nourished, he can better resist infection and continue to take part in his usual activities.

The side effects of treatment for cancer include nausea, vomiting, a sore or dry mouth and throat, or a general loss of appetite. ■ The nutritionist helps to personalize a feeding program for your child, taking these effects into consideration. ■ Sometimes, other feeding methods are needed to help your child stay well nourished, such as intragastric feeding or total parenteral nutrition (see Chapter 13 for more details). ■ If you have any questions about your child's eating habits, ask your doctor or clinic nurse to arrange an appointment with the nutritionist.

School Teacher: Regular school attendance and maintaining your child's academic standing is vital. ■ Children who can't attend school for a long period of time may be entitled to a tutor, provided by the local school board. ■ There may be a school teacher in the hospital who provides individual or classroom lessons to students who are hospitalized. Working closely with the students' home schools, these teachers teach children in the hospital classroom or bedside, ensuring that the students remain as up to date as possible with the material being learned by their classmates. ■ If you child knows he will not have weeks of "catch-up" when returning to school, it can often help him deal with the stress of a long hospital stay. ■ During periods when your child may not be attending school, it's still important for him to keep contact with teachers, even if just to keep up to date on what his friends are doing.

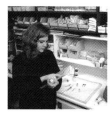

Clinical Pharmacist: Pharmacists answer questions about drugs and provide counselling to families attending the clinic. ■ As well, they may provide the following services:

• Preparing chemotherapy to be given in the clinic
• Scheduling and monitoring chemotherapy
• Giving medications, through an outpatient dispensary, along with the relevant cancer foundations/agencies
• Providing supplies needed to maintain right atrial catheters (see Chapter 7) through the outpatient dispensary.

Data Manager/Clinical Research Associate: The care of children with cancer is complex, and there are increasing numbers of children who survive their diseases. ■ As a result, there is an enormous amount of information generated. ■ Maintaining this information is usually the responsibility of the data manager/clinical research associate. ■ Much of this information is used by numerous research studies at pediatric cancer centers; your child may be participating in one or more of these studies. ■ A variety of samples (for example, blood and bone marrow) are obtained for these studies. ■ All of this information must be collected, organized, stored (confidentially), and analyzed.

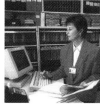

Clinic Secretary: The clinic secretary keeps complete, current, and easily accessible records on every child. ■ Efficient communication with other health professionals, especially your referring physician (usually your family doctor or pediatrician), is a vital part of this job.

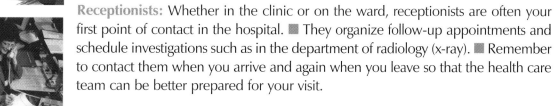

Receptionists: Whether in the clinic or on the ward, receptionists are often your first point of contact in the hospital. ■ They organize follow-up appointments and schedule investigations such as in the department of radiology (x-ray). ■ Remember to contact them when you arrive and again when you leave so that the health care team can be better prepared for your visit.

Other Health Care Workers: From time to time, the services of other specialists, such as physiotherapists and psychiatrists, may be needed. ■ They are members of our extended team and they provide important care. While many people play a part in your child's health care team, maintaining confidentiality relating to his care and that of your family is a high priority.

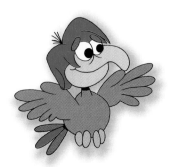
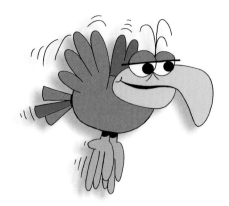

CHAPTER 2 IN BRIEF

You can take comfort in knowing that your child's health care team is dedicated to providing the best care possible. This team is composed of individuals highly trained in diagnosing and treating children with cancer. In charge of your child's care is the pediatric oncologist, a specialist in treating childhood cancer. A pediatric surgeon and radiation oncologist may be involved as well.

One nurse will be assigned as your guide and main contact throughout treatment and beyond. This nurse will help educate you and your child about cancer, its treatment, and side effects.

Child life specialists will look after the emotional well-being of your child and help prepare him for tests and treatments, while social workers will assist you and your family to function as best it can during this demanding time. Nutritionists will help keep your child well nourished to fight infection, keep up energy levels, and prevent major weight loss.

All of these people, along with many others, from pharmacists to physiotherapists, will take an active, important role in your child's treatment. If you have any questions or concerns, don't be afraid to ask. They are there to help.

NOTES

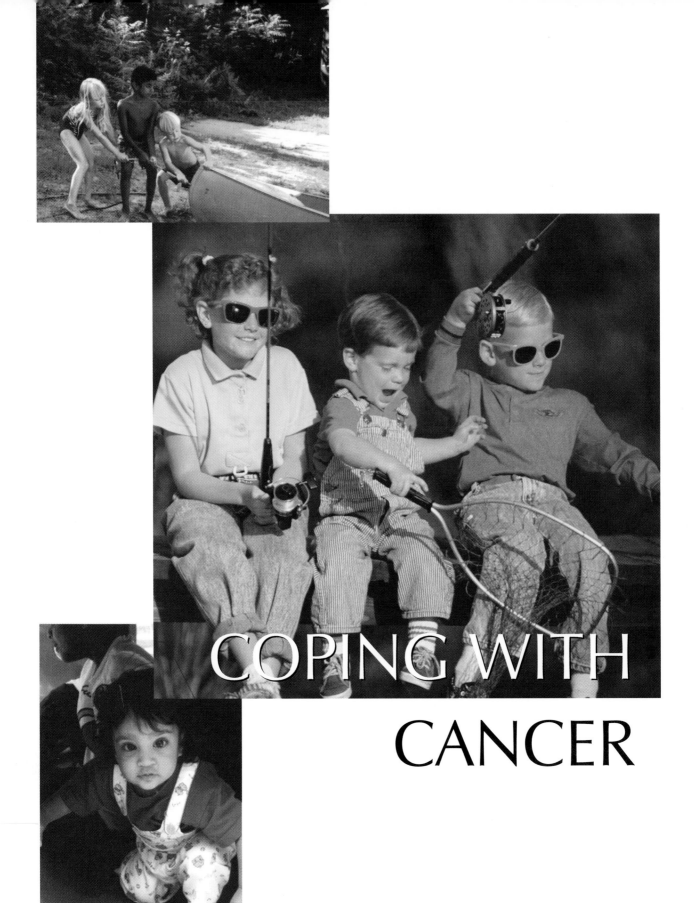

COPING WITH
CANCER

THIS SUBJECT WILL BE COVERED IN THREE PARTS: SUPPORT SYSTEMS, COMING OFF THERAPY, AND CARING FOR THE DYING CHILD.

Support Systems

There are many support services available for children with cancer and their families. Don't be afraid to ask for help! ■ Everyone can use extra help at some time during the course of treatment, whether it's emotional, financial, or anything else. ■ The social worker in your child's treatment team can help you find services for you and your child. ■ Listed below are some of the existing services that might be helpful.

Camps

• Camps offer residential, day, family, and leadership programs to children with cancer and their families at little or no cost. ■ These camps are available for present and former patients. ■ Experienced medical staff from the cancer treatment centers supervise the children's health care needs. Children with cancer and their siblings have the chance to meet, play, and share with children who have dealt with, or are dealing with, similar life experiences. ■ Learning new skills at camp increases their confidence and improves their self-image, giving them a greater sense of control and responsibility in their lives. ■ Many of the children and adolescents in camp programs are away from home for the first time. ■ The separation is often difficult for parents and children, but the great experience at the camp is usually worth it. ■ Be sure to ask the clinic staff about camp facilities in your area.

American and Canadian Cancer Societies

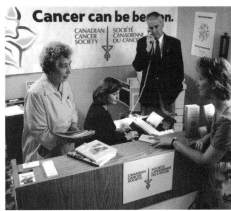

The American and Canadian Cancer Societies offer many support services for you and your child. ■ Below are some of the services that may be provided:

• Transportation from home to the cancer treatment center. ■ This may include transportation by a volunteer driver or help with the cost of public transportation.
• Help with the cost of non-professional care in the home, including homemakers and health care aides. ■ Help with the cost of non-professional child care is also available.
• Assistance with the cost of dressings and external medications.
• Support for the cost of drugs that control pain and discomfort.
• When medical equipment is not available free of charge, assistance with rental costs for a specified period of time.
• Financial assistance for the room and board of a family member or close friend who is needed to help care for a cancer patient during treatment, with the written request of a physician.
• Partial assistance for the purchase of wigs.

Be sure to contact your local Cancer Society branch to find out about these and other services.

American Red Cross/Canadian Blood Services

These agencies are well known for excellent blood donor clinics that keep hospitals supplied with blood products. ■ They can also provide useful information about bone marrow and blood stem cell transplantation. Local branches are listed in the telephone book.

Counselling

The hospital's social worker can provide short-term counselling during the course of treatment and can consult with child life and child psychiatry services available to you and your family. ■ As well, the social worker can refer you to services closer to your home.

Fulfilling Wishes

Wish foundations fulfill the wishes of children who have a life-threatening illness or are terminally ill. ■ They can help you make something pleasurable happen for your child. Please ask the clinic staff for the name of a wish foundation near you.

Government Assistance

Government departments—state/provincial and local—may offer financial assistance to help you meet the costs of transportation, drugs, and equipment needs of a disabled child. ■ "Handicap" and "disability" may be defined as limitations on activities of daily living. ■ Government programs may also provide professional services including a visiting home nurse, physiotherapist, speech therapist, or occupational therapist. ■ Check with your social worker about these benefits in your state/province or community.

Ronald McDonald House

This is a temporary home for parents whose children are critically ill. ■ There is a small fee for the use of this facility. If you wish to register at the House, please speak with the clinic staff.

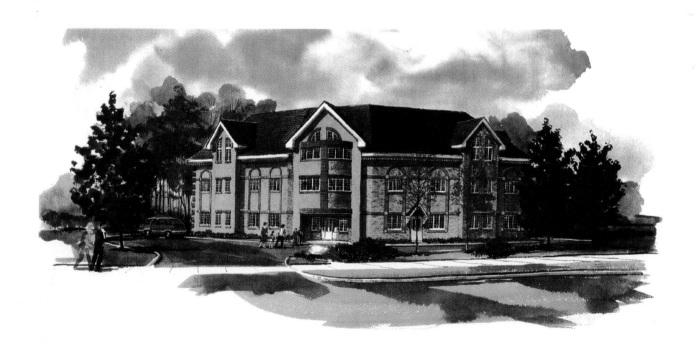

14

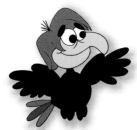

Support Groups

There are many groups available to the families and children who are having cancer treatment. ■ These groups provide children and their families with the opportunity to share ideas, concerns, and information with others who are in similar situations. ■ Some of these groups are listed below. ■ For more specific information, please ask a clinic staff member.

Parents' Support Group/Parents' Advocacy Group

Support groups are available to parents wanting to share and learn from their common experiences of having a child with cancer. ■ Many parents have found them to be helpful in coping with, and understanding, many of the complex issues surrounding cancer. ■ Some of the topics that have been discussed are

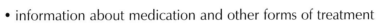

- information about medication and other forms of treatment
- dealing with the school system
- handling other children in the family
- concerns about discipline
- long-term survival
- insurance and employment prospects.

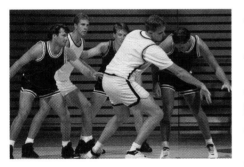

Adolescent Groups

Adolescence is a time of remarkable growth and change—both physical and emotional. ■ Adolescents start to become more independent of their family and form ideas of their own. ■ The opinions of their friends and peer groups are often more important. ■ The teenager with cancer goes through the normal changes of adolescence as well as dealing with a life-threatening illness. ■ Friends are important in adolescence, so this is a key time to offer teenagers a group where they can discuss and share their ideas and feelings about cancer with other teenagers. ■ Groups for adolescents may be run by hospital staff, but the teenagers are responsible for deciding on topics they wish to discuss. ■ Topics discussed often include

- the effects of treatment on lifestyle
- handling the side effects of medications
- being treated differently from others
- how to cope with changes in physical appearance
- dealing with family issues.

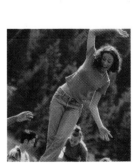

The adolescent group may be attended by teens on and off therapy.

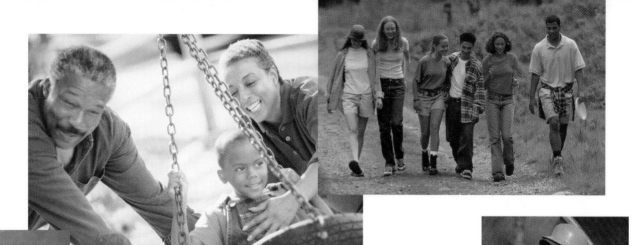

School-Age Children

The school-age child looks toward his friends and adults outside the family to measure his self-worth. ■ It is an age that relies heavily on his being "one of the gang." ■ He enjoys games and roles and needs to achieve status, both at school and with his friends. ■ The disruption created by illness often means many visits to the hospital. ■ Fortunately, there are many opportunities to foster interaction, communication, and support for children in this group. ■ A school visit can be arranged with the clinic nurse, child life specialist, and social worker. If he wants, your child may go along too.

Preschool Children

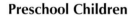

Preschoolers begin to need independence and control. ■ They need to interact with other children at this age, and play becomes a very important part of life. ■ They use play in a variety of ways— to learn about their environment, themselves, and social relationships—and gradually develop skills through drawing, building, and painting. ■ These children like to dress up and pretend to be a mother, father, baby, doctor, nurse, firefighter, and so on. ■ This allows them to try out different ways of behaving, hide some of their anxieties, and understand their feelings.

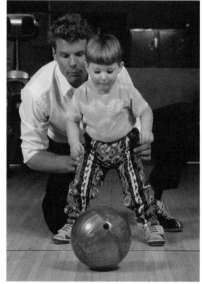

By using activities and medical play with both school-age and preschool children, child life specialists help children with their growth and development and assist them in coping with the challenges of cancer.

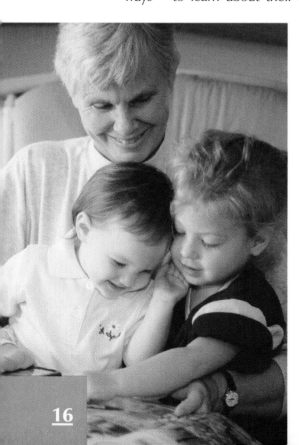

16

Coming Off Therapy

Due to advances in treatment, more and more children are completing therapy and being cured of cancer. ■ Reactions to coming off therapy vary with the age of the child, and those reactions may differ between a child and his parents.

Although the period of treatment may be difficult, families recognize that the drugs are fighting against cancer and prevent it from coming back. ■ So, as therapy comes to an end, they may be afraid. ■ In particular, parents and older children may worry about the cancer returning. ■ This anxiety is normal, but you may need help from the clinic staff to cope with it. ■ Talk about it directly and honestly. ■ Other help, such as religion, can play an important role in reducing anxiety. ■ Some parents and children find formal support groups useful at this time. ■ Regardless of your child's or family's reactions, it is important to realize that the clinic staff and services are still available to you even though treatment will soon be over.

The highest risk period for the return (recurrence) of cancer varies with the specific disease. ■ Rest assured that your child will continue to be watched for signs of the cancer returning, physical growth and development, and progress in school and other activities. ■ Follow-up visits may include examination of blood, urine specimens, x-rays, and other tests, depending on the nature of the original disease. ■ The length of time between visits will be extended as time goes on, providing there is no sign of the cancer returning. Eventually, your child will require only once-a-year visits.

As clinic visits become less frequent, you may lose contact with staff and perhaps other families and friends attending the clinic. ■ This may cause you and your child to feel insecure and anxious. ■ During this time, some people feel a loss of special status; others welcome it. ■ The clinic staff recognize that the end of therapy is a significant time of change, and they are available to make this period of adjustment easier for you and your child.

Coming off therapy is the time to review with your child's physician any and all of your concerns around treatment, outlook (prognosis), return of the cancer (recurrence), and long-term side effects.

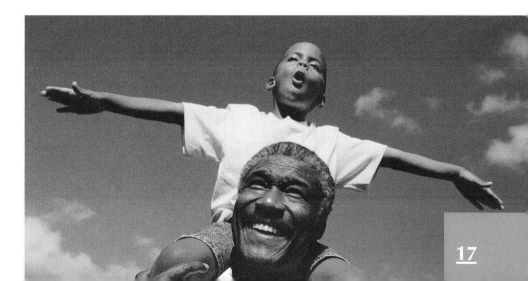

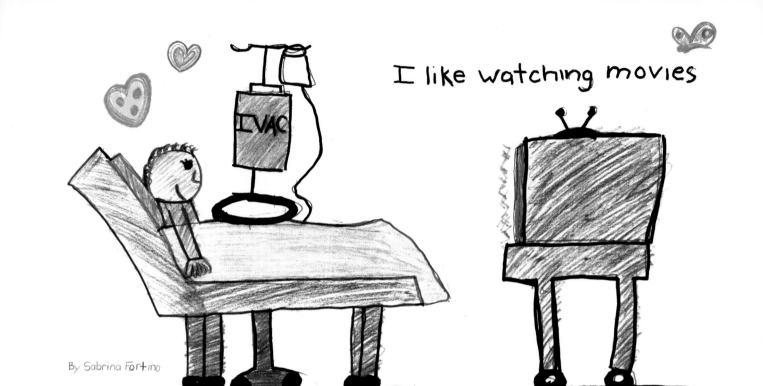

I like watching movies

By Sabrina Fortino

Care for the Dying Child

Unfortunately, there will be children whose cancer is advanced to a point where a cure is not possible. ■ At this time, the side effects of treatment may be worse than any benefits of continuing with aggressive therapy. ■ This is the time when the parents and health care team must take the difficult step of changing their focus from cure to ensuring the best quality of life for the dying child. ■ There are many aspects to this care (called palliative care), which are discussed below.

Physical Comfort. Parents are concerned that their child will suffer pain when he is dying. ■ Fortunately, there are medicines that effectively control all types of pain. ■ For most children, pain control can be achieved at home by the family. ■ This requires a close working relationship between the family, child, and health care team. ■ If at any time the child's pain needs medications through a vein (intravenously), he can be admitted to the hospital where the pain is controlled quickly. ■ After that, pain control can be continued at home.

Nausea, vomiting, and bleeding can often be controlled easily at home. ■ Intravenous fluids and antibiotics (to manage dehydration and infections), blood transfusions, and nutritional support may also be given at home, when possible.

Psychological Well-Being. A child's understanding of, and reaction to, dying are mostly age related. ■ Children under five years of age have great anxieties about evil and darkness and separation from loved ones. ■ Many of these children don't understand the finality of death and believe it can be reversed. ■ Remaining within the support of the family is the greatest comfort for the child. ■ Older

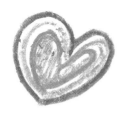

children, between the ages of six to nine, better understand the permanence of death and fear the pain and suffering that may be involved. ■ By discussing these anxieties with his family and the clinic staff, a child is often able to achieve a certain sense of acceptance and peace. ■ Adolescence is a period of great change and altered body image at puberty. ■ It is the beginning of independent decision making and the increasing importance of peer acceptance. ■ There may be extreme swings of behavior from dependence to withdrawal to aggression as the adolescent attempts to balance these changes. ■ This age group may benefit most from being able to discuss their fears with their parents, peers, and the clinic staff.

Honesty. One of the many difficult tasks facing parents is talking honestly and openly to their child who is dying. ■ What is said will depend on the age of the child and the particular religious and cultural influences in the family. ■ Remember that honesty with the child is extremely important. ■ Secrecy places tremendous strain on the child, who is usually aware that his care has changed and who knows of other children who have become as sick as he is and have died. ■ The child is often afraid to ask about dying and death because his parents haven't been able to talk about it. ■ This silence denies the child the chance to express his emotions, concerns, and questions. ■ Often, many of the child's greatest anxieties can be eased simply by talking about them.

Family Considerations It is a personal decision about where the child is best cared for while dying and at the time of death. ■ The clinic staff will provide support no matter which decision the family makes. ■ The most comforting place for the child is usually in his home, in his own room with his family and friends. ■ Provided that the child's problems, such as pain or nausea, can be well controlled at home and that the parents are physically and emotionally able to care for him, this setting is the most comforting for the child. ■ However, there may be times when a short or long stay in hospital will help the child and his family. ■ This is not a sign of failure or of poor care provided at home; a dying child is a constant concern and a physical and emotional strain. ■ If the child does come into the hospital, he and his family are given as much privacy as possible. ■ Intrusion by hospital staff is minimized, and visitation by friends can be restricted by the family. ■ The activities of the ward are reduced so there is the least disturbance to the child's peace. ■ No matter where a dying child is cared for, the clinic staff will do their best to continue support from the hospital, clinic-based health workers, and community groups. ■ Their flexible approach means that most problems can be handled in either the home or hospital setting, based on maintaining the quality of life of the child and family, according to their circumstances and beliefs.

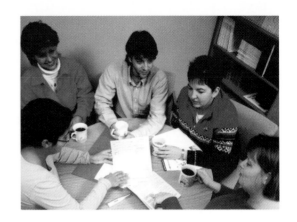

Many families have other children, and it's hard to know how to involve the other children in the care of the dying child. ■ Again, the healthy child's age will determine how much he understands. ■ It's often difficult to accept that a child is dying. ■ Parents and siblings will find themselves under a great deal of stress that may cause tensions between spouses and bad behavior in the healthy children. ■ It's important to recognize that each person is grieving and to accept support from friends and clinic staff.

The relationship between parents and their children is often the most intense relationship of life. ■ The death of a child leaves parents with many strong, different feelings. ■ A self-help group of bereaved parents can be extremely helpful in sharing, supporting, and learning.

The death of a brother or sister throws the family into a turmoil. ■ Parents who are trying to deal with the death of one child may not have much energy left over for the other children. ■ It may also be the first time that the other children in the family have come across death. ■ Talking with others who have gone through similar experiences can help the surviving children better understand themselves and their parents.

The death of a child is the most devastating event imaginable. ■ There is no shame in needing help to walk through the valley of this shadow. ■ Perhaps this help will come from a family member, a friend, another parent, or a team member. ■ Seek it wherever you may find it. The health care team would like to help.

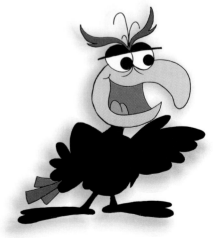

CHAPTER 3 IN BRIEF

Help Is at Hand

There are several support systems in place to help you and your family cope during the diagnosis and treatment of cancer. Whether you have emotional, financial, or other problems, there is always someone to lend a helping hand – cancer societies, wish foundations, assistance and support programs, and summer camps, to name a few. Ask the clinic staff for more details. Remember, admitting you need help is a sign of strength, not weakness.

The End of Therapy

Relief is a normal reaction when your child's therapy is drawing to a close. But, believe it or not, so is anxiety and fear. You and your child might worry about the possibility of cancer returning, and you might miss the regular contact with, and attentions of, the clinic staff. If you or your child feel anxious, talk to a member of the health care team. They can help you contend with this time of tremendous change.

The Prospect of Death

While the cure rate for childhood cancer is high, there are some children whose cancer can no longer be treated. At this time, enhancing quality of life for your child becomes the primary goal. Much can be done, even at home. The age of your child will determine how much and what information to provide about death. Above all, it is essential to be honest and open, so that your child can ask questions and talk over his fears. The death of a child is devastating for you and your family. Don't endure the pain alone. Seeking help – be it from a friend or member of the health care team – can make all the difference.

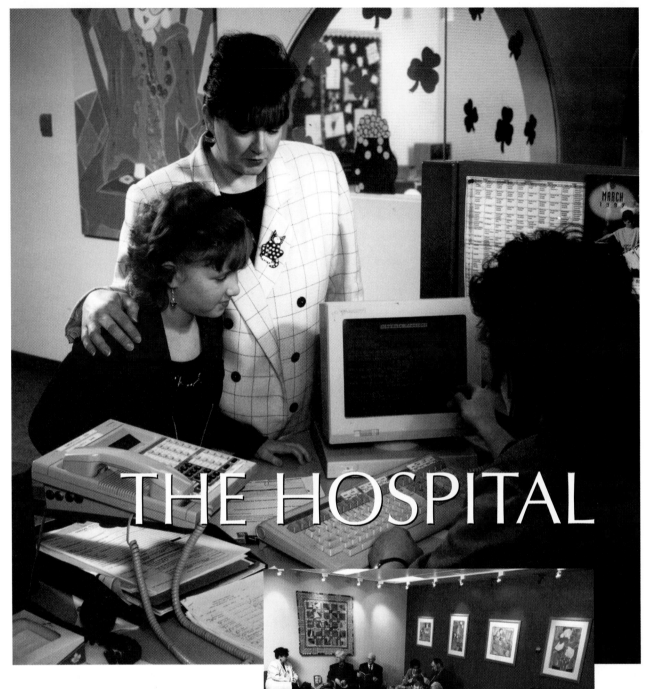

THE HOSPITAL

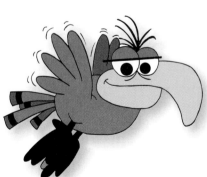

YOUR CHILD WILL HAVE BEEN ADMITTED TO THE
HOSPITAL TO DIAGNOSE HIS ILLNESS AND DETERMINE
A SUITABLE TREATMENT PLAN.

The First Admission

This process may take several days and will include specific blood tests, x-ray examinations, and other investigations depending on your child's illness. ■ The staff will explain any tests as they arise and will keep you informed of the results. ■ When a diagnosis is made, one of the physicians will discuss it with you, explaining in detail your child's disease and the treatment plan. ■ Explanations will take place regularly as treatment progresses.

Accommodation

Rooms are usually assigned on the basis of medical need. ■ For example, if a child has a low white blood cell count (neutropenia) or a contagious infection, he may be given a private room. ■ If he is receiving chemotherapy, he will not need a private room and may be put in a semi-private room.

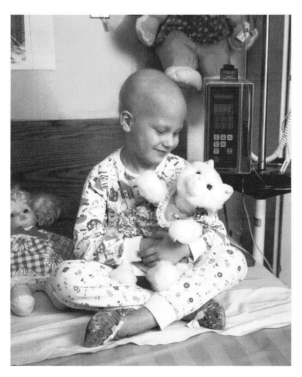

In many hospitals, a cot is provided in each room so that one parent may stay with the child. ■ Please fold up the cot daily so that morning care can be provided for your child.

If you do not wish to sleep in the room with your child and are from out of town, there may be a Ronald McDonald House that can provide accommodation. ■ Talk to the social worker to arrange this, if necessary.

You may bring things from home for your child's room, but please don't leave the room in a cluttered state. ■ We need to ensure that it is safe and accessible for cleaning.

Ward Routines

The nurses who will care for your child on the wards have special training in pediatric

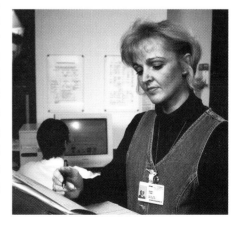

oncology. ■ They receive a report about your child as soon as they come on shift. ■ To provide the best care for your child, the nurses must always receive this report. ■ Unless the problem is urgent, please understand that a response to your request at this time may be delayed until the report is completed.

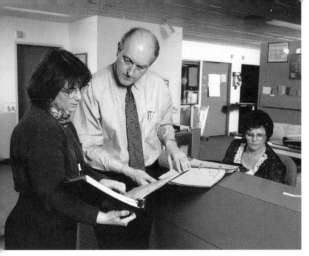

Ward Rounds

Normal rounds take place every day. ■ The hematology-oncology health care team will meet to discuss the patients and any new issues that have come up in the previous 24 hours. ■ Usually, after rounds, the team will update you and answer any questions you may have. ■ If you miss the team, please ask your ward nurse if you have any questions. ■ She will be aware of the issues discussed and will ensure that your questions are answered by the right person.

Meals

Meals are delivered at regular times. ■ Check with your nurse for the exact time. ■ A nutritionist is available to talk about menu options. ■ Any food brought in from home should be properly labelled and stored in the fridge. Please remember to remove personal items from the fridge when your child leaves the hospital.

Blood Sampling

Blood sampling is usually done in the morning, with results normally back around noon. ■ The physician will discuss the results of these and other tests with you after the ward rounds.

Playroom

The playroom hours are posted on the door of the playroom. If your child's white blood count is too low (neutropenia) or chemotherapy is in progress, he can't go to the playroom. ■ Child life staff can spend some time with your child in his room while he is isolated. ■ A teen room may be available for the older children.

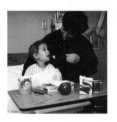
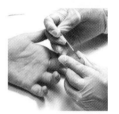
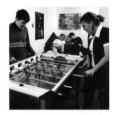
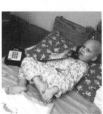

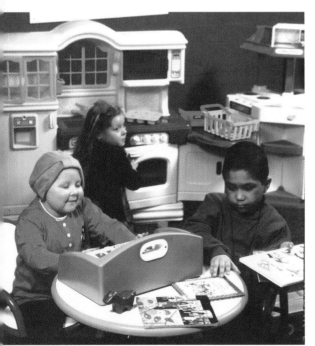

For safety reasons, children with intravenous pumps should stay in the areas close to the ward or playroom. ■ See your child's nurse to arrange for some time off the ward when this equipment is not required.

Telephone

Each room has a telephone. ■ Phone calls will be directed there, and you can ask to receive calls directly. ■ Questions about a child's condition will only be answered if received from the parents. ■ Please ask family members to speak to you about your child's condition.

Television/VCR/Video Games/Computers

Each room usually has a small television. ■ There are VCRs and video games available for patient use. ■ The equipment is for all patients on the ward. ■ Nursing staff do not monitor its use. ■ TVs and VCRs from home are not allowed in the hospital for electrical safety reasons. ■ Computers with modems may be available for patient use.

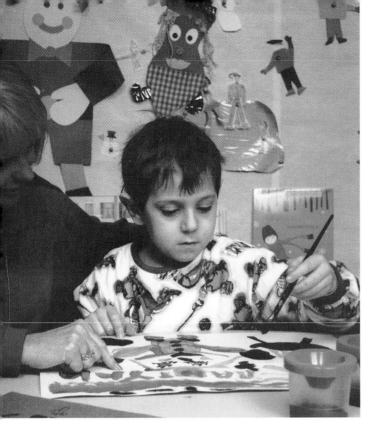

School

There may be a school room in the hospital, staffed by teachers from the local board of education. ■ If your child is of school age and well enough, he will be encouraged to go to the classroom. ■ If he is isolated in his room, but well enough to do some school work, the teacher will spend time with him in his room. ■ The school teacher assigned to your child can also speak with the teacher at your child's own school.

Further Admissions

After treatment has started, your child may need to be admitted again to hospital for specific therapy or to manage a complication, such as an infection that needs intravenous antibiotics. ■ Often he will be isolated in a private room to protect him from getting a second infection and to prevent his infection from spreading to another child. ■ Your child won't be able to play with other children until the infection is under control and his blood counts recover.

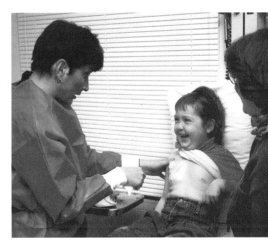

Blood products are usually given in the outpatient clinic, but an admission to hospital may be necessary. ■ Some children will be admitted to hospital when long-term chemotherapy is needed or when nausea and vomiting are a problem and more easily controlled by intravenous medications. ■ Surgery also requires hospitalization. ■ Children who are dying may need to be admitted to treat symptoms such as pain or nausea.

Planning for Discharge

A plan of treatment is needed when your child is ready to leave the hospital. The home care co-ordinator will be told of your child's special needs, and arrangements may be made for a nurse to visit your home to provide care. ■ A schedule will be drawn up for you to bring your child to the outpatient clinic for a follow-up visit and continued therapy.

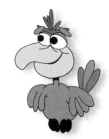

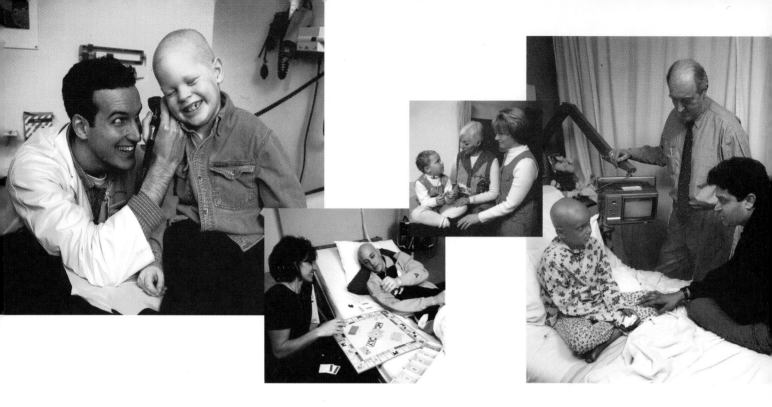

CHAPTER 4 IN BRIEF

Children don't like to be in hospital. They're away from home, being poked and prodded, and encountering many strangers. Facing one of the most difficult experiences in their young lives, children often feel helpless. As a caring, loving parent, you play a fundamental role in helping your child to cope.

Creating a comforting environment for your child is probably a priority for you. We will do what we can to help. It's true that hospitals have rules – rules that facilitate high-quality care in a safe environment. But they can be flexible to accommodate your needs and those of your child. For instance, you may sleep in the same room as your child, and favorite toys or special foods can be brought from home.

Your health care team will work hard to treat you and your family the way they would want to be treated. But please keep in mind that meeting the medical needs of your child must always come before your personal preferences.

NOTES

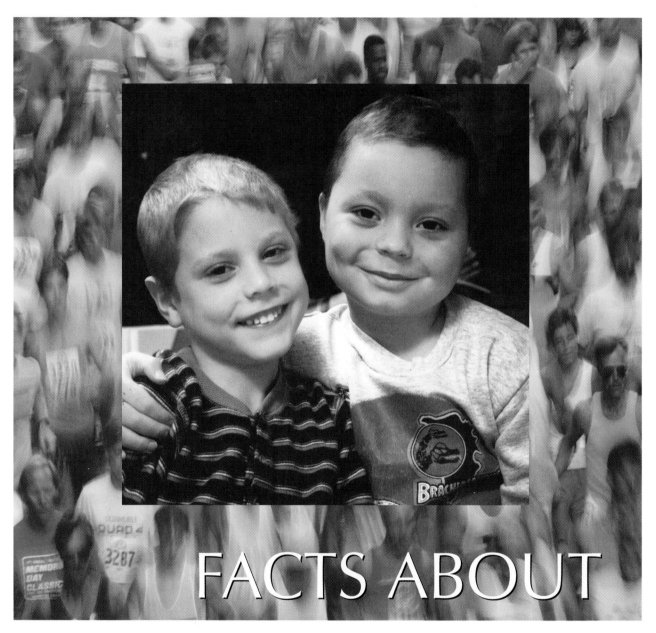

FACTS ABOUT
SPECIFIC DISEASES

SINCE THIS BOOK IS MORE ABOUT PEOPLE THAN DISEASES, ONLY A LIST OF THE MOST COMMON CANCERS IN CHILDHOOD IS INCLUDED IN THIS CHAPTER.

You will receive much more information about the specific cancer your child has. ■ Each type of cancer in this chapter is covered in six sections.

What is it? The nature of the cancer and its causes (if known) are discussed, as are its various types (if relevant), for these relate to different treatments and prospects of cure.

Who gets it? How often the cancer occurs, the most common ages affected, and patterns of inheritance (if any) are described.

Where is it? The original site(s) of the cancer with major symptoms and physical signs and local and distant (metastatic) spread of the cancer are listed.

How is it found (and measured)? Tests used to make the diagnosis and to follow the child's progress through treatment and beyond are explained. ■ A detailed program tailored to your child's cancer is provided separately by your health care team.

What is the treatment? General aspects of treatment are considered. ■ Details about an individual cancer will be given separately by your health care team.

What are the chances of cure? The prospects for permanent recovery, according to each category of cancer, and the outcome following a return (recurrence) of disease are presented. ■ Please remember that these are averages; information particular to your child will be provided by your child's oncologist.

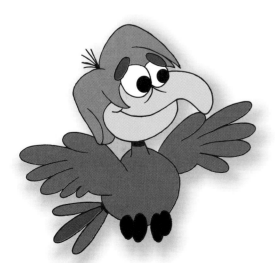

The following types of cancer are described:
- Acute lymphoblastic leukemia
- Acute myeloid leukemia
- Hodgkin's disease
- Non-Hodgkin's lymphoma
- Neuroblastoma
- Wilms' tumor (nephroblastoma)
- Rhabdomyosarcoma
- Osteogenic sarcoma
- Ewing's sarcoma
- Central nervous system tumors: medulloblastoma, astrocytoma/glioma, and ependymoma
- Retinoblastoma
- Germ cell tumors (including teratomas)

ACUTE LYMPHOBLASTIC LEUKEMIA (ALL)

What is it? This is a form of cancer that starts in the white blood cells (the lymphocytes). ■ These cells are produced in the bone marrow (the soft part inside bones) and circulate in the blood. ■ There are two major kinds of lymphocytes—T cells and B cells—that help protect the body from foreign substances. ■ In leukemia, the lymphocytes are poorly developed and can't do the work of the mature white blood cells. ■ The leukemia cell grows and multiplies in an uncontrolled manner and crowds out normal blood cells.

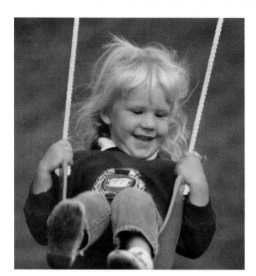

Who gets it? ALL accounts for one quarter to one third of all cancers in children. ■ It affects about one child in 2,000 and occurs most commonly around the age of four years. ■ Like other forms of cancer, ALL is not contagious and is seldom inherited, although the healthy identical twin of a child with ALL has a greater chance of having the disease. ■ Children with Down's syndrome or some other rare congenital disorders (existing since birth) are much more likely to develop ALL than are healthy children.

The cause of leukemia is unknown. ■ Exposure to chemicals, such as benzene, and large doses of radiation may lead to leukemia.

Where is it? The disease begins in the bone marrow and spills over into the blood. ■ Other parts of the body that normally contain many lymphocytes, such as the liver, spleen, and lymph glands (nodes), become involved and enlarged. ■ When first diagnosed, the disease has already spread, even into the brain and spinal cord, although usually without symptoms and signs. Because the cancer cells replace normal blood cells in the bone marrow, the child has

- fewer red blood cells (anemia), seems pale, and feels unusually tired
- fewer white blood cells (neutropenia) and is more likely to develop serious infections
- fewer platelets (thrombocytopenia) and bruises and bleeds easily.

When ALL spreads from the bone marrow into the solid bone, a child often feels pain in his limbs.

How is it found (and measured)? A simple blood test can tell doctors that ALL may be present, but other tests, including examination of the bone marrow, are needed to make a definite diagnosis.

What is the treatment? A combination of drugs is given by mouth and by injection into a vein (intravenously), into a muscle (intramuscularly), and into the fluid that surrounds the spine (intrathecally). ■ Some children also receive radiation therapy to the head.

What are the chances of cure? Children who have standard-risk ALL enjoy a 90 percent prospect of permanent recovery from the disease. ■ Those who have high-risk ALL have a 70 percent chance of cure. ■ Most children who have a return of the cancer (relapse) can be treated again successfully in the short term and will have no detectable disease (remission). ■ But many will have further relapses and eventually die of this disease. ■ For a small minority who have had a relapse, bone marrow transplantation may provide a cure. ■ After seven years of freedom from ALL, relapses are rare.

ACUTE MYELOID LEUKEMIA (AML)

What is it? This form of cancer usually starts in the white blood cells (granulocytes/ neutrophils or monocytes). ■ These cells are produced in the bone marrow and circulate in the blood. ■ The cancer cells continue to have many of the features of normal granulocytes or monocytes. ■ Some of these cells are more immature than others. ■ The cancer cells multiply in an uncontrolled manner and crowd out normal blood cells in the bone marrow.

Who gets it? AML accounts for about one fifth of all leukemia in children. It affects about one child in 10,000 and occurs most commonly in teenagers. ■ Like other forms of cancer, AML is not contagious and is seldom inherited, although the healthy identical twin of a child with AML is at considerable risk of also having the disease. ■ Children with Down's syndrome or some other rare congenital disorders (existing since birth) are much more likely to develop AML than are healthy children.

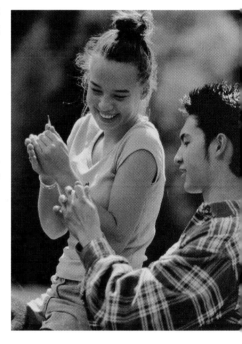

Where is it? The disease begins in the bone marrow and spills over into the blood. ■ Other parts of the body that normally contain many granulocytes and monocytes, such as the liver and spleen, become involved and enlarged. ■ When first diagnosed, the disease is already widespread.

Because the cancer cells replace normal blood cells in the bone marrow, the child has
• fewer red blood cells (anemia), seems pale, and feels unusually tired
• fewer white blood cells (neutropenia) and is susceptible to serious infections
• fewer platelets (thrombocytopenia) and bruises and bleeds easily.

When AML spreads from the bone marrow into the solid bone, a child often feels pain in his limbs.

How is it found (and measured)? A simple blood test can tell doctors that AML may be present, but other tests, including examination of the bone marrow, are needed to make a definite diagnosis.

What is the treatment? A combination of drugs is given by mouth and by intravenous injection. Sometimes drugs are also given into the fluid that surrounds the spine (intrathecally).

What are the chances of cure? Children who have AML have up to a 50 percent prospect of permanent recovery from the disease. ■ For the minority of children who have a suitable donor, bone marrow transplantation offers the best hope for cure. ■ Most children who have a return of the cancer (relapse) can be treated again successfully in the short term and will not have detectable disease (remission). ■ But many will have further relapses and eventually die of this disease. ■ For a small minority who have a relapse, bone marrow transplantation may provide a cure.

HODGKIN'S DISEASE

What is it? This is a form of cancer called malignant lymphoma. ■ It is a disease that starts in the lymph glands (located in areas such as the neck, armpit, and groin) and can spread throughout the body through the lymphatic system. ■ There are four main types of Hodgkin's disease. ■ The cause of Hodgkin's disease is unknown.

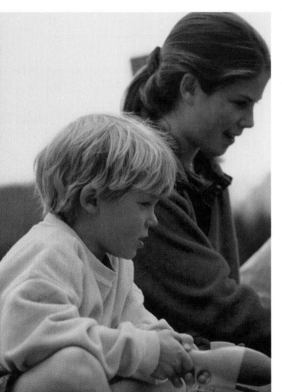

Who gets it? Hodgkin's disease occurs in approximately one child in 10,000 and is rare in children under the age of five years. ■ There is no evidence that this cancer is inherited.

Where is it? The disease appears to begin in one or more of a group of lymph glands, most commonly in the neck. ■ These glands become swollen—usually the first symptom that prompts a visit to the doctor. ■ Often the cancer is limited to a small number of closely related glands. ■ In 50 percent of children it spreads to the chest. The abdomen may also be involved. ■ In the minority of children, there is a high fever, weight loss, and night sweats. ■ These symptoms are more common if the cancer is extensive and are associated with the need for more aggressive treatment and a poorer outcome.

How is it found (and measured)? Removing an enlarged lymph gland usually means that Hodgkin's disease can be easily diagnosed. ■ Many tests, especially x-ray examinations, are then done to see the extent of the cancer and plan the best therapy. ■ This process is known as staging.

What is the treatment? Children whose cancer is limited to a small area (stage 1) may be treated only with radiation therapy to the affected area of the body. ■ In children with more extensive (stage 2 or 3) cancer, a combination of chemotherapy and radiation is used. ■ In children with widespread (stage 4) disease, the main form of treatment is intensive chemotherapy.

What are the chances of cure? The prospect of cure for children with stage 1 or 2 disease is approximately 90 percent and is greater than 50 percent even for those with widespread (stage 4) disease. ■ There are many side effects of treatment (see Chapter 7 for more details). ■ A small number (perhaps 5 percent) of children who receive chemotherapy for Hodgkin's disease will develop another form of cancer, such as acute myeloid leukemia. ■ Those children who experience a relapse of the original cancer often respond to further treatment, particularly if they received radiation therapy only.

NON-HODGKIN'S LYMPHOMA (NHL)

What is it? This is a form of cancer called malignant lymphoma. ■ It is a disease that starts in the lymph glands and can spread throughout the body by way of the lymphatic system. ■ There are two types of non-Hodgkin's lymphoma (NHL): lymphoblastic and non-lymphoblastic. ■ The causes of NHL are unknown.

Who gets it? NHL occurs in approximately one child in 10,000, usually between the ages of 7 and 11 years. Children who have rare problems with their immune systems have a greater chance of developing NHL. ■ There is no evidence that this cancer is inherited.

Where is it? In most children, NHL is already extensive when first diagnosed; about one third appear to start in the neck or chest, one third in the abdomen, and one third elsewhere. ■ There is often pain and swelling at the site of the cancer. ■ Other symptoms include abdominal bloating, weight loss, change in bowel habit, and fever. ■ If the chest is involved, there may be swelling of the veins in the head and neck and difficulty in breathing. ■ In about one third of the children, the cancer spreads to the bone marrow, brain, or spinal cord.

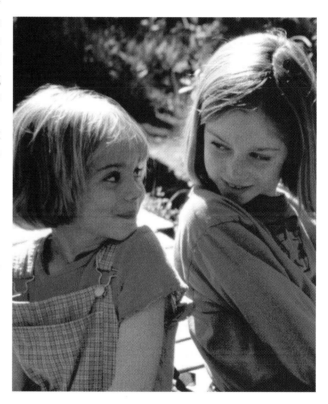

How is it found (and measured)? Diagnosis is usually made by removing an enlarged lymph gland, examining the chest by x-ray, or examining the abdomen through surgery. ■ Many tests, especially x-rays, are then performed to see the extent of the disease and plan the best therapy. This process is known as staging.

What is the treatment? Chemotherapy with combinations of drugs is the usual treatment. ■ Children with extensive NHL may need masses of the cancer removed by surgery if it is causing blockage in the intestine or may need radiation of large glands that are squeezing vital structures such as the windpipe. ■ Since many children with NHL have large tumors at the start of treatment, special care must be taken with their water and salt balance, and other medications may be needed to protect the kidneys from the chemicals released by dying tumor cells.

What are the chances of cure? The prospect of cure for children with NHL has improved considerably in recent years. ■ It is now approximately 70 percent overall. ■ A return of the cancer (relapse) after two years from the time of diagnosis is uncommon if the child has been free of the disease in the meantime. ■ Some children who have a relapse may be able to have bone marrow or blood stem cell transplantation.

NEUROBLASTOMA

What is it? This is a tumor made up of nerve cells that starts in the adrenal glands (which sit on top of the kidneys) or in nervous tissue that runs alongside the spine. ■ Most tumors are in the abdomen, half of these being in one of the adrenal glands. ■ Tumors may begin at more than one place in the same child. ■ Of all forms of human cancer, neuroblastoma is the one most likely to be cured without treatment.

Who gets it? This is one of the most common solid (non-leukemic) tumors in children, affecting approximately one child in 7,000. ■ Almost all children with neuroblastoma are under the age of five years at diagnosis, with about 50 percent being under the age of two. ■ There is no evidence that this cancer is inherited.

Where is it? Normal nerve cells, from which neuroblastoma may develop, are located anywhere, from the neck to the pelvis. ■ Since the structures where neuroblastoma starts lie deep within the body, the tumor is often very large when it is diagnosed. ■ This cancer may be noticed in the following ways:

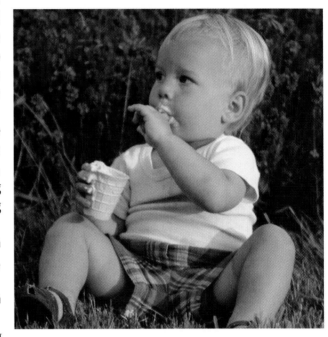

- The expanding tumor can be seen (in the abdomen, for instance) or it puts pressure on neighboring normal structures. ■ For example, the tumor may be in the chest, causing breathing problems, or in the pelvis, causing bowel or bladder problems.
- The tumor interferes with the normal function of the nerve from which it started. For example, muscles in the eye might be paralyzed.
- The tumor produces too many hormones, which may cause diarrhea and high blood pressure.
- If widespread, it may affect the skin (appearing as bluish lumps) or bone (resulting in pain).

In contrast to most other cancers, neuroblastoma seldom spreads to the lungs. Unfortunately, many patients who have this tumor have widespread disease by the time it's diagnosed.

How is it found (and measured)? Neuroblastoma is usually diagnosed by looking at the abdomen during surgery or by x-ray. ■ Many tests are then done to see the extent of the disease and plan the best therapy. ■ This process is known as staging. ■ The blood and urine are also tested for substances produced by the tumor; the amount of these substances tells how much cancer is present.

What is the treatment? For patients whose cancer is limited to a small area (stage 1 or 2), surgically removing the tumor is often the only treatment needed. ■ Chemotherapy, with or without radiation therapy, will be needed when the cancer is more extensive.

What are the chances of cure? Children who have stage 1 or 2 neuroblastoma completely removed by surgery alone have a very high chance of cure. ■ But the outlook is poor for most children who have widespread disease at diagnosis. ■ In a special category of patient with neuroblastoma, the original disease has spread to liver, skin, or bone marrow (but not to bone). ■ These are usually infants, and about one third of them will be cured without treatment.

WILMS' TUMOR (NEPHROBLASTOMA)

What is it? This is a type of cancer of the kidney that is rare in adults. ■ There are two types of Wilms' tumor: favorable and unfavorable. ■ The response to treatment and prospect of cure are different for both types. ■ Most children with Wilms' tumor have the favorable type.

Who gets it? The disease affects approximately one child in 10,000, and most of them are less than five years of age when the diagnosis is made. ■ In a few cases, the disease is inherited from one of the parents.

Where is it? Since the tumor begins in one of the kidneys (organs that lie deep in the abdomen), it is usually large by the time the cancer is noticed. ■ It is often found by chance. ■ Symptoms include vague abdominal pain, high blood pressure, and passage of blood in the urine. ■ But, usually, the child is well. ■ Although the tumor is often large, it isn't usually widespread. ■ In particular, spread to the bones is rare. ■ Occasionally, both kidneys are involved.

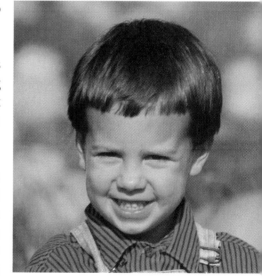

How is it found (and measured)? An accurate diagnosis is made by surgically removing the affected kidney. ■ Examining the abdomen at the same time will let the doctors see the extent of the cancer and plan the best therapy. ■ This process is known as staging.

What is the treatment? Children who have Wilms' tumor that is totally within the kidney and completely removed by surgery need only a short course of chemotherapy. ■ If the disease has broken out of the kidney, radiation therapy to the abdomen in combination with chemotherapy may be needed. ■ For a few children with widespread disease or disease of the unfavorable category, more aggressive chemotherapy is needed.

What are the chances of cure? Overall, the outlook for children who have Wilms' tumor is very good, and the great majority are cured. ■ However, for the children who have extensive or widespread disease and for those in the unfavorable category, the prospect for cure is less and may be no better than 50 percent.

RHABDOMYOSARCOMA

What is it? This is a form of cancer that starts in skeletal muscle (muscle found mainly in the limbs and trunk). ■ There are four types of rhabdomyosarcoma. ■ The outlook is good for children with the most common type. ■ The causes of this tumor are unknown.

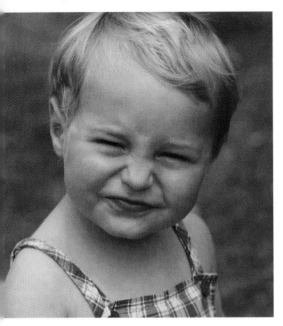

Who gets it? Rhabdomyosarcoma occurs in about one child in 20,000. ■ About 70 percent of affected children are less than 10 years of age, with most being between the ages of two and five years. ■ There is no evidence that this cancer is inherited.

Where is it? The first sign of rhabdomyosarcoma is usually a lump; the most common place is in the head and neck area. ■ If the cancer spreads, lymph glands, lung, bone marrow, brain, and spinal cord may be involved.

How is it found (and measured)? Diagnosis is made by removing part or all of the lump (depending on location) for careful examination under a microscope. ■ Many tests, especially x-ray examinations, are then done to see the extent of the cancer and plan the best therapy. ■ This process is known as staging.

What is the treatment? Until recently, the major forms of treatment were surgery and radiation treatment. ■ When the tumor was large or in a place not easily accessed, the child was often left with a major disability. ■ Completely removing the tumor by surgery is still the best treatment, if removing the tumor is straightforward, and is a good option for the child. ■ In these children, no radiation is needed. ■ When some tumor remains after surgery, radiation is used. ■ All children with this disease are given chemotherapy to get rid of tumor cells that may have spread before treatment was started. ■ If the cancer is extensive at the time of diagnosis or surgery is hard to perform, chemotherapy is used first to reduce the total amount of the cancer. ■ The rest is removed surgically and then radiation is given.

What are the chances of cure? For most children with rhabdomyosarcoma limited to a small area, the chances of cure are excellent (more than 90 percent). ■ The outlook for children with more extensive disease depends mainly on site and type of disease. ■ It ranges from poor (the prospect of cure being remote) to cautiously optimistic (the prospect of cure being about 50 percent). ■ After two continuous years of freedom from this cancer, the likelihood of its return (relapse) is low. ■ When a relapse does take place, only a few children will survive long term.

OSTEOGENIC SARCOMA

What is it? This cancer starts in bone, where the cancer cells produce abnormal bone-like material. ■ There are several types of osteogenic sarcoma. ■ In most instances, the cause of this cancer is unknown, although it can start in an area that has been given radiation before, usually when treating another type of cancer.

Who gets it? Osteogenic sarcoma usually affects adolescents—about one teenager in 20,000. ■ There is no evidence that this cancer is inherited.

Where is it? This tumor most commonly affects the bones around the knee and sometimes the shoulder. ■ Most children first complain of pain where the cancer is located but have no injury you can see. ■ The lungs are the most common organs to be affected if osteogenic sarcoma spreads.

How is it found (and measured)? In most instances, an x-ray examination of the painful area will show a tumor. ■ A definite diagnosis is made with a biopsy (tissue cut from the tumor during surgery). ■ Many tests, especially more x-rays, are then done to see the extent of the disease and plan the best therapy. ■ This is particularly important if amputation (cutting off) of a limb is to be avoided.

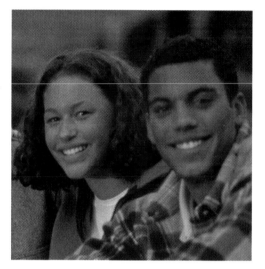

What is the treatment? Chemotherapy is the first choice of treatment for osteogenic sarcoma. ■ This reduces the size of the tumor, making it easier for the surgeon to save the limb and replace the affected bone with a normal or artificial bone. ■ Chemotherapy also immediately attacks any hidden cancer cells that may have spread and is continued to eliminate any remaining cancer.

What are the chances of cure? The prospect of cure has improved dramatically in the past 10 years. ■ Now more than 50 percent of all children with osteogenic sarcoma can look forward to being free of disease. ■ The return (relapse) of this cancer after three years is uncommon. ■ When spread to the lungs does occur, the outlook may still be hopeful if the tumor in the lungs is removed and further chemotherapy is given.

EWING'S SARCOMA
What is it? This cancer starts in or close to bone, but we don't know for certain which cells it comes from. ■ It can be difficult to tell Ewing's sarcoma apart from other cancers that involve bone. ■ There is no known cause of this cancer.

Who gets it? Ewing's sarcoma mainly affects adolescents—about one teenager in 50,000. ■ It is especially rare in blacks. ■ There is no evidence that this cancer is inherited.

Where is it? This tumor most commonly affects the thigh bone but may occur almost anywhere. ■ Pain, without any obvious injury, is the most common first symptom. ■ The disease can spread to the lungs, lymph glands, or other bones.

How is it found (and measured)? An x-ray examination of the painful area will show that a tumor is present. ■ A definite diagnosis is made with a biopsy (tissue surgically removed from the tumor). ■ Many tests, especially further x-rays, are then done to see the extent of the cancer and plan the best therapy.

What is the treatment? The affected part is removed by surgery only when the removal of the whole tumor has acceptable results for the child. ■ Amputation (removal of a limb) is usually not acceptable. ■ If removal of the complete tumor isn't possible, a combination of radiation therapy and chemotherapy with multiple drugs is used.

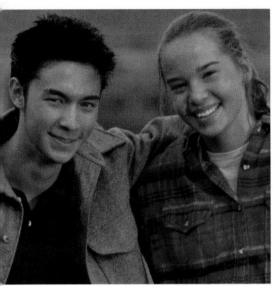

What are the chances of cure? More than 50 percent of patients with Ewing's sarcoma will be cured. ■ It is not common for this cancer to return (relapse) after three years. Relapses may be treated successfully with radiation therapy and drugs. ■ Children with Ewing's sarcoma may develop another type of bone tumor in the area where radiation therapy was given.

CENTRAL NERVOUS SYSTEM TUMORS

What are they? These are tumors that start in the brain or, less commonly, the spinal cord. Sometimes the cancer cells may come from nerve cells or, more often, from cells that support or cover the brain and spinal cord. The causes of these tumors are unknown.

Who gets them? As a group, central nervous system tumors are the second most common form of cancer in childhood, affecting about one child in 4,000. ■ The most common type of these tumors is medulloblastoma, followed by astrocytoma and ependymoma. Children in the five- to 10-year age group are affected most often. There is no evidence that these tumors are inherited.

Where are they? Since most of these tumors start in the brain, there is increased pressure within the skull. This can cause morning headache, vomiting, visual problems, fits (seizures), and changes in the way a child acts. ■ Medulloblastoma and cerebellar astrocytoma often create difficulties with balance, since they commonly begin in a part of the brain that controls this function. ■ Both medulloblastoma and ependymoma may spread down the spinal cord, and medulloblastoma may even spread outside the nervous system.

How are they found (and measured)? A definite diagnosis is made by removing part or all of the tumor by surgery and examining it under a microscope. ■ Tests, mainly CAT and MRI scans, must be done to see the extent of the cancer.

What is the treatment? By itself, surgery can cure some tumors, like cerebellar astrocytoma. ■ However, it is usually not a cure for others like ependymoma. ■ For these tumors, radiotherapy can be effective treatment. ■ Chemotherapy is not as good but is often used in very young children to delay or avoid radiotherapy.

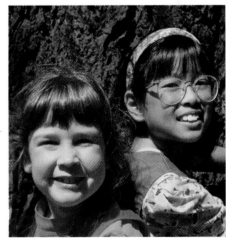

What are the chances of cure? If a cerebellar astrocytoma can be removed completely, the five-year survival rate is over 80 percent. ■ In medulloblastoma, about 50 percent of patients

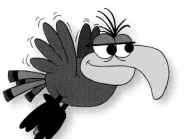
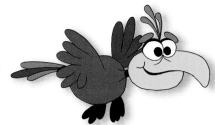

survive five years. ■ The outcome for ependymomas varies according to site of disease and microscopic features of the tumor but may approach a 50 percent survival at five years in the best circumstances.

RETINOBLASTOMA

What is it? This cancer begins at the back of the eye, from the cells that form part of the retina. The cause is unknown.

Who gets it? Retinoblastoma mainly occurs in very young children, most often before the age of two years. ■ It affects approximately one child in 20,000. ■ The tumor is often inherited, especially when it affects both eyes. ■ If one parent has had this disease, the risk for each child is about 50 percent.

Where is it? Retinoblastoma is usually limited to the eye, but multiple tumors may be present. ■ The most common first sign of this cancer is a cat's eye reflex, in which the pupil (the center of the eye) appears white instead of black. ■ The child may also have a squint in the affected eye. ■ If the tumor spreads outside the eye (this is uncommon), bone, bone marrow, or the fluid surrounding the brain and spinal cord may be affected.

How is it found (and measured)? A tumor can be seen by carefully looking at the back of the eye with a special instrument (an ophthalmoscope). ■ It can also determine whether more than one tumor is present and if both eyes are involved. ■ X-ray examination, including CAT scans of the skull, will tell if the disease has spread outside the eye. ■ It is important to know the full extent of the cancer, as that will decide the best treatment.

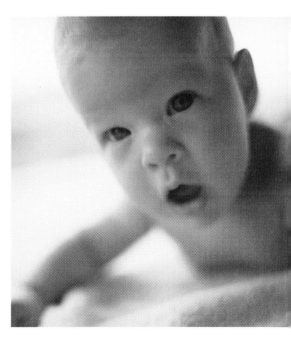

What is the treatment? It may be necessary to remove the affected eye or the more affected eye if both are involved. ■ When the tumors are small in size and number, radiation therapy or newer strategies are used. ■ The role of chemotherapy in treating retinoblastoma is being assessed.

What are the chances of cure? Even if both eyes are involved, the chances of long-term survival free of disease are better than 80 percent. ■ However, the amount of useful sight left after radiation therapy will vary from one child to another. ■ Children who receive radiation for retinoblastoma may develop bone tumors close to the eye.

GERM CELL TUMORS (including teratoma)

What are they? These are tumors that start in cells that have existed since we developed from a fertilized egg. ■ There are several types of germ cell tumors including dysgerminoma, seminoma, immature teratoma, endodermal sinus tumor, choriocarcinoma, or embryonal cell carcinoma. The best treatment and outcome depend on the type of germ cell tumor.

Where are they? The tumor usually appears in the abdomen but may begin anywhere, including an ovary. ■ In boys, the main location may be in a testis. ■ Swelling, with or without pain, is the most common symptom. ■ If the tumor spreads outside the abdomen, it is found most often in the lungs.

Who gets them? This group of tumors affects about one child in 40,000. ■ It is rare for a preschool child to be affected. ■ There is no evidence that this cancer is inherited.

How are they found (and measured)? A definite diagnosis is made by removing the swelling. ■ The surgeon must also see if the removal is complete or if there are other tumors in the abdomen. ■ A variety of tests, including blood tests, are done to determine the extent of disease.

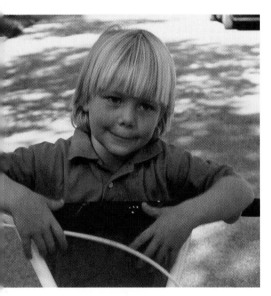

What is the treatment? For all children with germ cell tumors, it is important to remove as much tumor as possible by surgery. ■ Then radiation therapy is given to children with dysgerminoma or seminoma but not to those with the other disorders. ■ Children also receive chemotherapy with multiple drugs.

What are the chances of cure? The prospect of cure depends on the extent of disease, but even when a large amount of the tumor remains after surgery, there is a better than 50 percent chance of cure with chemotherapy (with or without additional radiation therapy).

CHAPTER 5 IN BRIEF

There are many types of childhood cancers, each with its own characteristics, treatment, and prospect of cure. Details on some of the major childhood cancers are covered in this chapter. Your health care team will provide you with more detailed information on the specific cancer your child has, how it will be treated, and what the outcome will be. If you're unclear about anything you're told or want to know more, be sure to ask. The more you learn about your child's cancer, the less overwhelmed you will feel.

NOTES

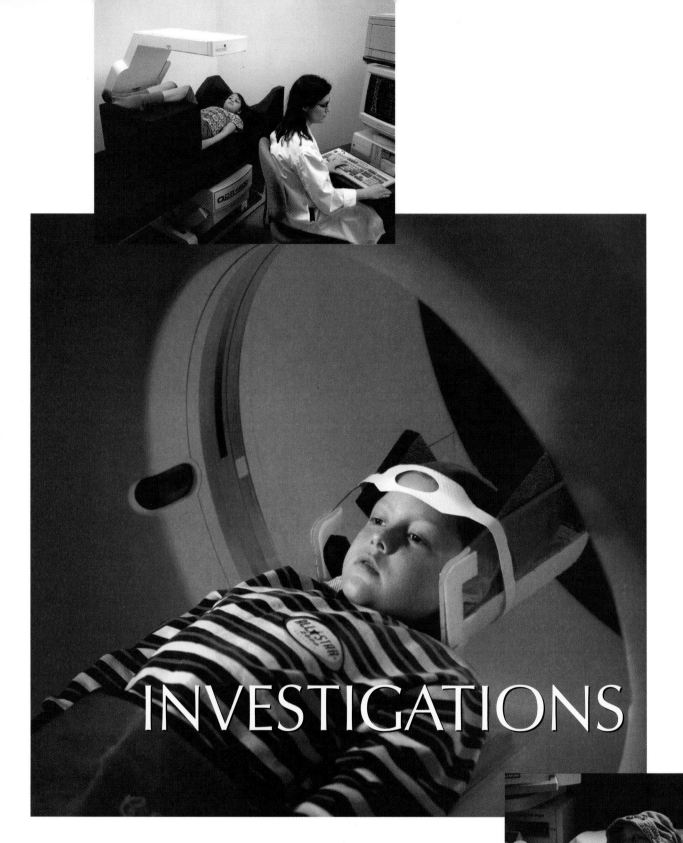

INVESTIGATIONS

IF A CHILD IS THOUGHT TO HAVE CANCER, MANY TESTS ARE DONE TO DETERMINE A DIAGNOSIS, THE EXTENT OR SPREAD OF THE DISEASE, AND THE BEST TREATMENT.

Many of these tests will be done regularly to see how the cancer is responding to treatment and to keep a watch on any side effects.

At first, most of these tests will be done when your child is an inpatient at the hospital, but afterwards many of them can be done safely on an outpatient basis. ■ Each test will be explained to you and your child by a member of the staff. ■ The very young child will need time with the child life staff in order to understand many of the tests. ■ The older child will need simple, clear explanations. ■ Your written consent may be needed for some tests.

The following section describes the types of tests that may be performed. ■ Keep in mind that not every test is needed for each cancer.

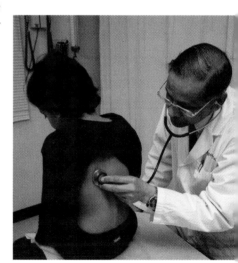

Index of Tests

Frequent
- Physical examination (physical, check-up)
- CBC (complete blood count)
- Urinalysis and blood tests of kidney function
- Liver function tests
- Checking vital signs (temperature, pulse rate, blood pressure, respiratory rate)

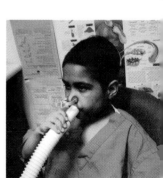

Infrequent
- Audiometry
- Bone marrow examination: Aspiration and biopsy
- Cardio-respiratory function
  - Echocardiogram
  - Electrocardiogram
  - Pulmonary function tests
- Electroencephalogram
- Electromyogram
- Lumbar puncture
- Tumor markers

- Radiology
  - Chest x-ray
  - Computerized axial tomography (CAT scan)
  - Barium studies: Barium meal, barium enema
  - Lymphography
  - Magnetic resonance imaging (MRI)
  - Myelography
  - Nuclear medicine (radioisotopic) studies
  - Ultrasonography
  - Angiography

Frequent Tests

Physical Examination (physical, check-up)

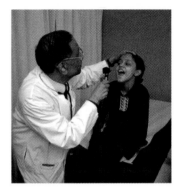

On most visits to the clinic, a doctor will do a physical examination to check your child's general state of health and to ask about any new problems. ■ Be sure to tell the doctor about any new symptoms such as colds, diarrhea, pains, fevers, rashes, or anything at all that has changed. ■ Most people find it useful to write down questions or problems as they arise so they're not forgotten.

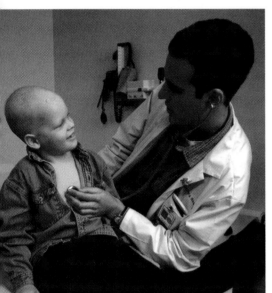

The doctor will then look in your child's eyes, ears, and mouth. ■ The neck, armpits, and groins will be felt for glands. ■ The heart, lungs, and abdomen are also examined. ■ In boys, the genitalia are examined from time to time. ■ Special attention will be paid to any areas of concern.

The physical examination takes only a few minutes and will not usually be uncomfortable for your child. ■ The doctor will discuss what he finds with you immediately and may have the findings confirmed by another doctor. ■ Occasionally, help may be needed from other health specialists such as dermatologists, neurologists, gynecologists, cardiologists, or respirologists. ■ If this is the case, your child may be seen either in the pediatric oncology clinic or elsewhere in the hospital/clinic.

Complete Blood Count

A complete blood count (CBC) is performed almost every time your child is at the clinic for treatment or follow-up exams. ■ The small amount of blood is used to measure the hemoglobin, white blood cell count (Lkcs or leukocytes), differential leukocyte count (diff), and platelet count.

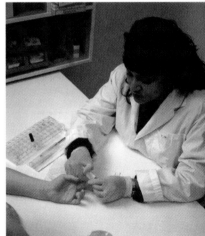

Blood may be taken by pricking your child's finger or, when other blood tests are needed, it may be taken in the clinic by inserting a needle in his vein (venous sampling). ■ Results from a CBC may take 30 minutes or more to obtain.

It's important to prepare your child for this test. ■ If he's afraid, the child life staff can help. ■ There is a brief, sharp pain from a finger prick, but this goes away quickly, with no longer-term side effects.

The hemoglobin refers to the amount of red pigment in the blood, which is responsible for carrying oxygen to each and every cell in the body. If it is too low, your child is anemic. ■ Signs of anemia include tiredness, weakness, and pale skin.

There are different kinds of white blood cells in the body; the most important are neutrophils, lymphocytes, and monocytes. ■ These white cells are necessary for fighting infection and maintaining immunity. ■ If the total white cell count or the

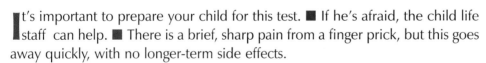

neutrophil count is too low, your child has a greater chance of getting an infection. ■ If this is the case, the clinic staff will advise you on what to do.

Platelets are needed for blood clotting. ■ If their count is too low, your child can bruise or bleed easily.

Urinalysis and Blood Tests of Kidney Function

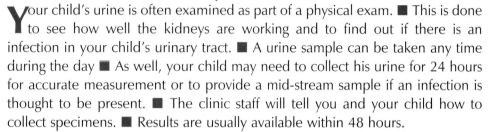

Your child's urine is often examined as part of a physical exam. ■ This is done to see how well the kidneys are working and to find out if there is an infection in your child's urinary tract. ■ A urine sample can be taken any time during the day ■ As well, your child may need to collect his urine for 24 hours for accurate measurement or to provide a mid-stream sample if an infection is thought to be present. ■ The clinic staff will tell you and your child how to collect specimens. ■ Results are usually available within 48 hours.

Blood tests are also used to measure how well the kidneys are working. ■ These tests measure salts such as sodium and potassium and products of protein breakdown such as urea and creatinine. ■ These tests also look for other substances, like calcium, magnesium, phosphate, glucose, and uric acid, which can tell how treatment is affecting your child's body.

Liver Function Tests (LFTs)

The liver is one of the most active organs in the body. ■ To find out how well the liver is working, there are certain tests that can be done on your child's blood at the time of diagnosis and regularly throughout treatment. ■ How often these tests are done depends on the type of cancer and the treatment your child is receiving.

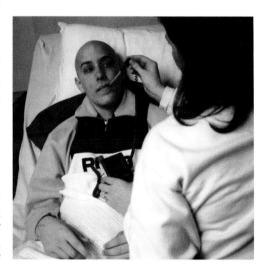

Checking Vital Signs (Temperature, Pulse Rate, Blood Pressure, and Respiratory Rate)

During clinic and hospital visits, your child will have his vital signs checked. ■ If an infection is thought to be present, or when chemotherapy or transfusions of platelets or red cells are given, more frequent checking of your child's vital signs may be needed.

Infrequent Tests

Audiometry

Your child's hearing will be tested to see if there is any hearing loss caused by treatment with certain antibiotics or anti-cancer drugs. ■ There is no specific preparation for this test, but we do need your child's cooperation. ■ The child life staff will explain, through

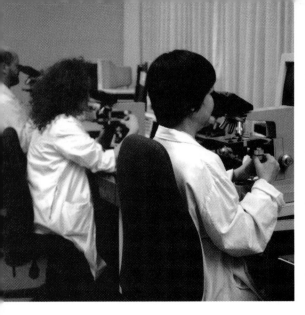

play, what the test will be like. ■ The testing is done in the audiology clinic and is tailored to the age of the child. ■ There are no side effects.

Bone Marrow Examination: Aspiration and Biopsy

The bone marrow is found in the center of bones. ■ It is the factory where blood cells are made. ■ Certain types of cancer may start in the cells of the marrow (e.g., leukemia, lymphoma) or may spread there from other places (e.g., neuroblastoma). ■ For these cancers, samples of the bone marrow must be obtained and examined. ■ The marrow is usually taken from the large pelvic or hip bone.

The test is usually done in the clinic or on the ward, where it takes about 15 minutes. ■ Sometimes, it must be done in the hospital's operating room.

Many hospitals now give short-term general anesthesia (given outside of the operating room) so that your child is asleep during the entire test and won't feel a thing. ■ Ask your health care team if this option is available at your child's hospital.

During the test, a needle is inserted into the bone, and a sample of marrow is withdrawn into a syringe (this is called aspiration). ■ A laboratory technologist may be present to prepare the jelly-like marrow so it can be examined under a microscope. Often, a second sample is taken at the same place using a different needle. ■ This second sample, termed a bone biopsy, is a small piece of hard bone tissue along with the marrow inside it. ■ Examining this material can provide more information about the cancer in the bone marrow.

The aspirated bone marrow will be ready for microscopic examination within a few hours, and the results will be available on the same day. ■ Bone biopsies take longer, and results are not usually available for 48 hours.

After the anesthetic wears off, your child will feel little or no aching or discomfort. ■ There are no long-term side effects of the aspiration or biopsy.

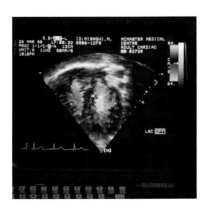

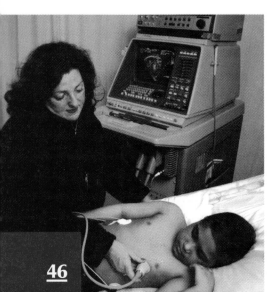

Cardio-Respiratory Function

A number of different tests, including an echocardiogram, electrocardiogram, and pulmonary function tests, are done in the cardio-respiratory department. ■ These tests tell the doctors about any side effects of treatment or any effects of cancer on the heart and lungs.

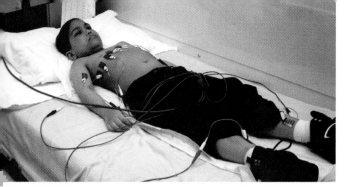

• Echocardiogram (Echo)

Using sound waves, an echocardiogram measures the motion of the walls of the heart and heart valves. ■ Your child must be able to lie quietly for the half-hour examination. ■ Sedation may be needed to help your child relax. ■ During the test, cold gel is put on the front of the chest, and a probe is passed back and forth over the skin covering the area of the heart. ■ The results are recorded on a TV monitor, which you and your child can watch. ■ When the test is over, your child's skin will be cleaned, and he will be able to return to normal activity. ■ There are no side effects.

• Electrocardiogram (EKG, ECG)

An EKG (ECG) records electrical activity of the heart, also showing how well it is working. ■ Again, your child must be able to lie quietly for about half an hour. ■ Rubber pads (called electrodes) are attached by wires to a machine (called an electrocardiograph) and are placed on his wrists, legs, and chest. ■ Recordings are made on a strip of paper for the physician to study. ■ There are no side effects, and your child will be able to return to normal activity after it's over.

• Pulmonary Function Tests (PFTs, Spirometry)

These tests measure how much air your child's lungs can hold and the strength and speed with which he can push air in and out. ■ During the test, your child will be seated and asked to take a deep breath. ■ Then a mouthpiece will be placed over his mouth, and he will have to exhale as fast as possible into the mouthpiece, completely emptying his lungs. ■ The mouthpiece is attached to a machine that will measure the volume of air and the force with which it is exhaled. ■ This will be repeated several times, with a rest between each test. ■ The test takes 10 to 15 minutes. ■ Sometimes, more lung function tests are performed on older children. ■ Your child may return to normal activity immediately following the test. ■ It has no side effects.

Electroencephalogram (EEG)

An EEG records the electrical activity of the brain on a machine (called an electroencephalograph). ■ It may be used to diagnose and/or test problems related to how the brain is working. ■ Generally, the test is done when the child is off medication for seizures, if this is possible. ■ The test will take about an hour. ■ During the test, your child will need to sit or lie quietly with his eyes closed. ■ Small electrodes are attached to his head or scalp with glue. ■ The glue washes out with shampoo. ■ There is no discomfort or side effects with this test. ■ Hair does not need to be cut. ■ The test results will be looked at by a physician (called a neurologist). ■ It may take several days for you to receive the results.

Electromyogram (EMG)

An EMG uses electrical stimulation to measure the activity in nerves and muscles. ■ In this way, the doctor will know how well they are working and will detect muscle weakness or abnormal sensations. ■ The test will take from an hour to an hour and a half and is done by

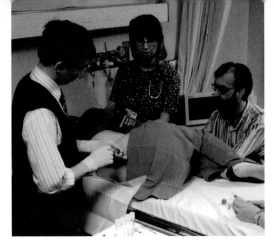

both a physician and a technician. ■ Electrodes are placed on the surface of the limbs, the peripheral nerves are stimulated, and the resultant electrical activity is measured. ■ Your child may feel some tingling sensation or at most a slight shock. ■ There are no side effects of this test, and the results will be available within 24 hours.

Lumbar Puncture (LP)

The brain and spinal cord (central nervous system) are surrounded by a clear, watery liquid called the cerebrospinal fluid (CSF). ■ The brain, spinal cord, and CSF are covered by a protective membrane. ■ Some cancers, such as acute lymphoblastic leukemia, may spread to the brain, spinal cord, or protective membrane. Taking samples of the CSF is one way to know if the disease has spread to these areas. ■ Many anti-cancer drugs do not pass from the bloodstream into the CSF, so some may be injected directly (intrathecally) into the CSF to stop cancer cells from growing in the central nervous system.

The way to obtain a sample of CSF is called a lumbar puncture (LP). ■ It usually takes place in the clinic or on the ward, although it may be necessary to do this test in the hospital's operating room.

Many hospitals now give short-term general anesthesia (given outside of the operating room) so that your child is asleep during the entire test and won't feel a thing. ■ Ask your health care team if this option is available at your child's hospital.

During this test, a needle is inserted between the vertebrae in the spinal column in the lower back (lumbar region). ■ The needle penetrates the protective membrane, the CSF drips out easily, and drugs can be injected through the needle if needed. ■ The results from the tests carried out on the CSF are usually available within a few hours.

After the test is done, it's important that your child lies flat for an hour or so to avoid developing a headache. ■ Still, a headache may develop later anyway. ■ Sometimes, there is a reaction in the protective membrane to the drugs injected, causing pain where the LP was done and even into the buttocks or down the legs. This pain can be helped by simple medications like Tylenol.

Tumor Markers

Some forms of cancer produce substances (called markers) that tell if the disease is present. ■ Finding and measuring these substances help make a more definite diagnosis. ■ Regular measurements can measure how much tumor is present and help determine how well treatment is working. ■ If a marker in the blood or urine reappears, it can be a valuable early sign of the return (relapse) of disease.

Radiology

X-ray pictures of parts of the body will be taken at the time of diagnosis and regularly after that to watch your child's treatment. ■ These tests are done in the radiology department.

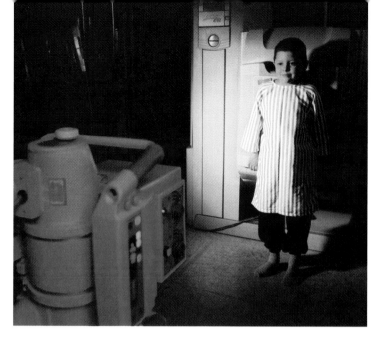

■ If you want to be with your child during x-ray examinations, you will usually be asked to wear a lead protective apron. ■ Pregnant mothers can't be near x-rays, so you should bring someone else to help if you are pregnant.

• **Chest X-ray (CXR)**

The chest x-ray looks at the lungs, heart, and bones making up the chest wall. ■ The test will take about 15 minutes. ■ If your child is under three years of age, he will be supported upright for the test in a device (called a Pigostat). ■ The Pigostat (named after its inventor) is a non-painful brace that holds your child still, in the right position, so that a clear x-ray can be taken. ■ Infants may be wrapped tightly in a blanket while the x-ray is being done. ■ An older child is examined standing, facing the film holder or the x-ray machine. ■ Sometimes, a mobile machine may be brought to your child's room to take pictures with him sitting up in bed.

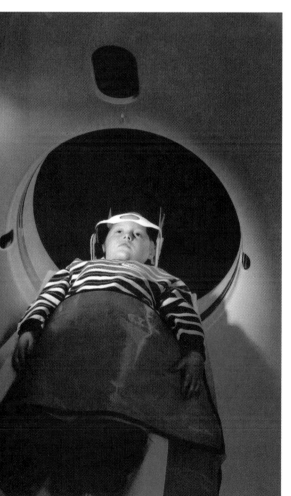

• **Computerized Axial Tomography (CT, CAT Scan)**

With CAT scans, a computer is used to put together a cross-sectional picture of the body from many images. ■ These scans are used for areas like the brain, spine, chest, abdomen, and pelvis. ■ The test usually takes a half to one hour. ■ Instructions about eating and drinking before the test will be given to you. ■ If your child is having a CAT scan of his abdomen and pelvis, he will not be able to eat or drink for several hours before the test, so that contrast dyes can be used. ■ Contrast dyes, given in juice or milk or through a vein, improve the quality of the pictures taken. ■ If your child has allergies, tell the radiologist or technician before the injection or swallowing of the dyes.

Your child must lie completely still, so sedation is sometimes needed to help him relax. He will pass through a large, circular machine that takes many pictures of the required area. ■ There are no side effects, except if your child is allergic to the contrast dye.

• Barium Studies

Barium meal examines the upper part of the digestive tract, including the esophagus (food pipe), stomach, and duodenum (part of the small intestine just below the stomach). ■ It will take about half an hour. ■ Your child must fast for several hours before the test. The x-ray technologist will give him a cup of barium (like a thick milkshake, but with a less pleasant taste) to drink through a straw and will explain when and how much to drink. ■ Your child will have pictures taken of him while lying on a table and while standing up. ■ After the test, he will be asked to drink lots of fluids to help clear the barium from his gut. ■ Stool passed for 24 to 72 hours after the test will be white. ■ Complications are rare from barium meals.

Barium enema examines the lower part of the digestive tract (the colon) and will take about an hour. ■ You will be told how to prepare your child at the time the appointment is booked. ■ Your child may need to take a laxative at home before coming to the hospital or may receive a cleansing enema in the radiology department. ■ He will lie down on his side while the barium is run into his rectum through a tube. ■ The room lights will be lowered so the radiologist can see the barium on a TV screen while your child is moved into many positions. ■ Pictures will be taken throughout the test. ■ It can be tiring and uncomfortable for your child. ■ Stool passed for 24 to 72 hours after the test will be white. Complications from barium enemas are rare.

• Lymphography

This test gives information about the condition of the lymph system and takes four to five hours to complete. ■ Your child must be able to lie still, so sedation may be needed to help him relax. ■ To help pass the time, he can bring along a book or game. ■ During the test, a contrast dye is injected into the feet. ■ Tell the physician about any allergies or reactions to drugs before the injection. ■ The dye is traced as it travels slowly to the chest, and x-ray pictures are taken. ■ More x-ray pictures are taken the next day to show the dye that remains in the lymph glands (nodes). ■ Your child may notice a bluish color in his urine and stool for 48 hours after the examination and some soreness at the place where the contrast dye was injected. ■ Other side effects are rare.

• Magnetic Resonance Imaging (MRI)

Magnetic resonance imaging uses a powerful magnet and radiowaves to scan the inside of the body without using x-rays. ■ This information is fed into a computer to give a detailed picture.

The test can take an hour or more. ■ Your child may need sedation so that he can relax and lie completely still. ■ If sedation is needed, your child can only have clear fluids by mouth from midnight up to several hours before appointment time. ■ From then to the time of the test, your child should have nothing by mouth. ■ There are no known side effects from an MRI.

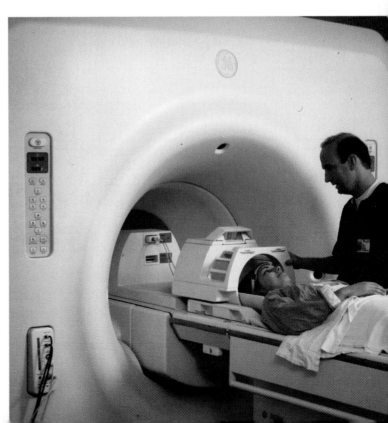

• Myelography

This test tells if there are cancer cells in the spinal cord and surrounding space. ■ The test usually is done on an inpatient basis only. ■ It will take about an hour. ■ Sometimes, a general anesthetic may be needed. ■ Your child may have nothing to eat or drink for at least eight hours before the test, and a line will be placed in his vein (IV line) to give sedation and to keep him hydrated for several hours following the test. ■ Instead of an IV line, a right atrial catheter (see Chapter 7) may be used.

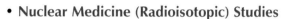

Your child will lie on a table. A lumbar puncture will be done, and contrast medium will be injected into the cerebrospinal fluid. ■ Tell the physicians about any allergies or reactions to drugs before the injection. ■ X-ray pictures will be taken while the table is tilted. ■ When he returns to the ward, your child will lie at a 45-degree angle for 24 hours. ■ This reduces the chances of developing a headache, backache, and nausea. ■ If these side effects do occur, they can usually be controlled by medication.

• Nuclear Medicine (Radioisotopic) Studies

By detecting radiation given off by a radioisotope, these studies provide information about organs like bones, liver, spleen, kidneys, brain, and lungs. ■ A solution, containing the radioisotope, is injected into a vein. ■ Sometimes a waiting period is needed before the isotope is taken up by the organ that is being studied. ■ With some scans, you and your child may have to return to the nuclear medicine department the next day to complete the test. ■ You will be given detailed information about the scan your child will have. ■ The radioactive isotopes are given in such small amounts that there is no danger to you or your child. ■ The level of radiation in this test is usually less than that of a chest x-ray and is mostly limited to a specific organ.

Some children will have a test to check the bone mineral content of the forearm and vertebrae (spine). ■ This is called a bone density examination. ■ No radioactive isotopes will be given. ■ Your child will need to lie quietly during the procedure.

• Ultrasonography

Ultrasonography is used to look at organs in the abdomen such as the kidneys, liver, spleen, and pancreas. ■ The test is done in the radiology department and will take about an hour. ■ The type of preparation will depend on the age of your child and the organ to be studied. ■ For instance, your child may not be able to eat solid foods immediately before the test. ■ The radiology staff will tell you how to prepare. ■ Ultrasound pictures are made from sound waves (which you can't hear) from a special vibrating crystal. ■ The test is usually done in a dark room. During

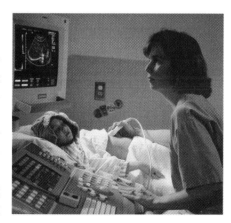

the test, warm gel is put on the part of your child's body to be scanned, and a probe is passed back and forth over the skin. ■ The technician will be watching the images on a TV monitor. ■ You and your child can watch too. ■ There are no known side effects of this test.

• **Angiography**

This test looks at the structure of blood vessels. ■ A contrast dye is injected directly into a blood vessel while rapid pictures are taken. ■ The contrast dye (as used in other scans such as CAT scan) is sent through a catheter, which is placed in the blood vessel (artery or vein) to be tested. ■ Serious complications of angiography are possible, including the cutting (perforation) of a blood vessel, excessive bleeding (hemorrhage), or blood clot (thrombosis) For more information about hemorrhage and thrombosis, see Chapter 8.

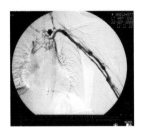

CHAPTER 6 IN BRIEF

Tests are useful tools for the health care team, providing vital information to plan the best care possible. This is why your child will undergo regular testing throughout his treatment and after its completion. Some tests are simple and straightforward, like blood and urine tests. Others are more complicated, such as CAT scans or ultrasounds. If your child is scared or uncomfortable about these tests, we can give him medication to relax or sleep.

For the most part, tests are painless. You'll be glad to know that specialized tests (like bone marrow exams and lumbar punctures), which used to cause some discomfort and distress, now are performed usually under a general anesthetic. Your child is asleep during the entire procedure and doesn't feel a thing.

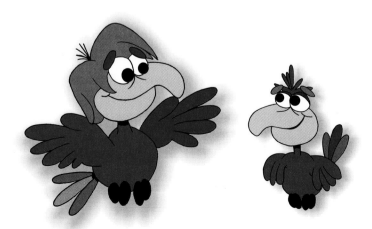

NOTES

6

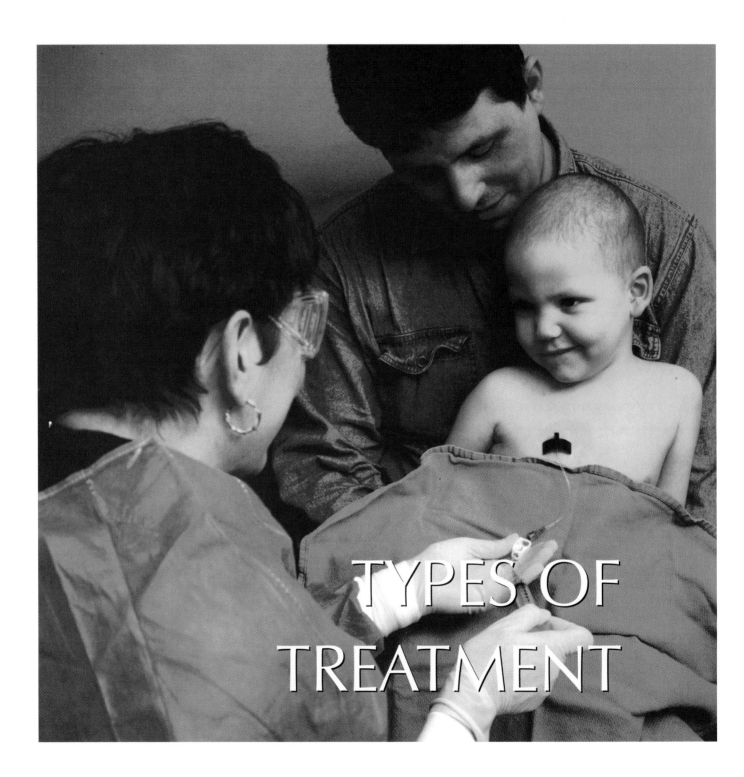

TYPES OF
TREATMENT

THERE ARE THREE MAIN WAYS IN WHICH
    CANCER IS TREATED: DRUGS (CHEMOTHERAPY),
SURGERY, AND RADIATION THERAPY.

Chemotherapy

While surgery and radiation therapy are used to treat cancer in a specific site or location, drugs travel in the bloodstream throughout the body and can treat cancer in many locations.

Drugs are given in several different ways.

Orally (By Mouth)

Some medications are given in tablet or capsule form. ■ The medication dissolves in the gut and is then absorbed. ■ For very small children, you may need to "split" tablets so that your child has the right dose. ■ If this is the case, speak with the pharmacist as some medications can be made into a liquid so that giving the right dose is easier.

By Injection

Many drugs are injected into a vein (intravenously). ■ Certain drugs can be injected into the tissue just under the skin (subcutaneously), while others need to be injected into a muscle (intramuscularly). ■ Sometimes drugs are given by another method if they need to go to a certain place, such as the spinal fluid (intrathecally).

How the Drugs Work

We're not entirely sure how some drugs kill the cancer cells. ■ In general, drugs stop cancer cells from growing or reproducing. ■ This is usually done by interfering with the cells' DNA (genetic material essential to the cells' reproduction) or a biochemical process. Unfortunately, normal, healthy cells are often affected at the same time. ■ These cells include those that line the mouth and intestines, skin (including hair), cells of the reproductive system (testicles, ovaries), and the bone marrow. ■ The effects on these healthy cells are often only temporary, and the healthy cells usually recover. ■ Remember, there is no relationship between the severity of side effects and how well treatment is working. ■ Many children respond well to treatment with only mild or moderate side effects.

Common Side Effects of Chemotherapy

While your child is likely to experience some side effects from his treatment, keep in mind that

- side effects are often temporary and, for the most part, go away after treatment has finished.
- there are treatments that can prevent some side effects.
- it is unlikely that your child will experience every side effect of every medication that he receives.

- Most children tolerate anti-cancer drugs better than adults do. This means that children can receive larger doses more often than adults. ■ In part, that's why cure rates for pediatric cancers are higher than for adult cancers.

Below are some of the common side effects of chemotherapy.

Mouth and Intestines

• **Nausea and vomiting:** Many anti-cancer drugs can cause nausea and vomiting. Fortunately, there are effective medications that can control and even prevent nausea and vomiting. ■ Called anti-emetics, these medications are given by mouth, or injection, usually before, during, and often for a day or two after chemotherapy. ■ If your child has nausea/vomiting, give him clear fluids and tell his doctor.

• **Loss of appetite; pain and sores (ulcerations) in the mouth:** Certain drugs cause changes in the sense of taste and smell. ■ Sores in the mouth (ulcerations) can also occur. If this happens to your child, don't force him to eat and drink. Instead, try to be flexible, and give him food he likes. ■ Changes in taste and smell usually don't last long. ■ Talk to the nutritionist about how you can deal with this problem. ■ If your child has severe ulcerations, he may not be able to take anything by mouth because of pain. ■ He may need to stay in hospital for a short time to control pain and obtain nutritional support. ■ Good care of teeth and gums is important throughout therapy. ■ Regular tooth brushing with a soft toothbrush is a good idea. ■ Children are often given an oral anti-fungal preparation and a non-alcohol-based mouth rinse. Avoid some commercial mouthwashes as they have a high alcohol content that can cause drying of the mouth and increase the pain from ulcers.

• **Constipation and diarrhea:** If your child is constipated, give him plenty of fluids and try a natural laxative such as prune juice. ■ If he has diarrhea, note the color and frequency of stools and give him clear fluids to drink. ■ Tell your child's doctor if there is frequent diarrhea, since this may lead to dehydration, especially in infants and young children. ■ Don't buy over-the-counter medication to treat diarrhea or constipation without asking your child's doctor first.

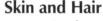

Skin and Hair

Certain drugs can leak from an intravenous injection and seriously harm local skin and deeper tissue. ■ Using a right atrial catheter, such as a Port-A-Cath or Hickman/Broviac, reduces the chances of this happening. ■ See Chapter 8 for more details.

Sometimes, your child may develop a rash. ■ Usually, this is not serious but may mean that your child is allergic to the drug. ■ Report all rashes to your child's doctor immediately.

Losing some or all hair is very common. ■ Chemotherapy affects all areas that have hair. Hair will grow back once chemotherapy is completed. ■ Usually, it takes six months or longer for the hair to grow back fully, although fine hair may start to grow back while your child is still on chemotherapy. ■ Losing hair is hard to accept,

especially for adolescents. ■ Planning ahead for hair loss can help. ■ Try matching a wig to existing hair or start a collection of hats and bandannas. ■ The clinic staff can help your child adjust to hair loss. ■ Be sure to talk to them.

Bone Marrow

Bone marrow forms all cells that circulate in the bloodstream. ■ Anti-cancer drugs can reduce the production of these cells, including

• **Red blood cells:** These cells carry oxygen throughout the body. ■ When there are too few red blood cells, anemia can result. ■ During these periods, your child may look pale, feel tired, and have little energy. ■ If the number of red blood cells falls too low, your child may need an injection of red blood cells. ■ This is called a transfusion.

• **Platelets:** These cells form a "plug" in blood vessels when we cut or injure ourselves and stop the bleeding. ■ When the number of platelets falls, your child may bruise and bleed more easily. ■ This may happen with only a minor injury or without an injury (such as nose bleeds). ■ A transfusion of platelets is often needed to keep the number of platelets high enough. ■ During periods when your child's platelet counts are low, he should stay away from certain activities like contact sports.

• **Neutrophils:** These are special white blood cells that fight infection. ■ When the neutrophils are lower than normal (neutropenia), your child will get infections more easily. ■ Unfortunately, neutrophils can't be given easily by transfusion like red cells or platelets, although certain hormone-like substances can stimulate their production. ■ Sometimes, certain anti-cancer drugs may produce a fever. ■ This usually occurs within 24 hours of your child receiving the drug and can be treated with medications like Tylenol. ■ However, it's important to immediately report to your child's doctor any fever of more than 38°C/100°F and any signs of infection. ■ See Chapter 9 for more details.

Your child's blood counts will be watched frequently. ■ With repeated chemotherapy, the bone marrow may take longer to recover. ■ If this is the case, there may be a delay in giving more chemotherapy, and the doses may need to be changed.

Muscles and Nerves

Some anti-cancer drugs may damage nerves. ■ Tingling, numbness, or a burning sensation in the fingers and/or feet may be a sign of nerve damage. ■ Your child may be clumsier than usual or may sometimes lose his balance. ■ He may also lose muscle strength. ■ These side effects usually go away, but it may take some time. ■ Physiotherapy may help. ■ Often, it's necessary to change the dose of the drug causing the side effects. ■ Some anti-cancer drugs, as well as certain antibiotics,

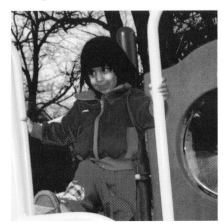

cause some hearing loss. ■ This is usually detected early through hearing tests (audiometry), and treatment is then changed. ■ Serious damage to the brain is rare, although there are often changes in a child's mood and behavior.

Urinary Tract

The kidneys filter out unnecessary or harmful waste products from the blood and get rid of them in the urine. ■ Many anti-cancer drugs can harm the kidneys or the bladder. ■ Radiotherapy in the area of the bladder may increase the harm caused by certain drugs. ■ As cancer cells are killed by anti-cancer drugs, large amounts of by-products are released. ■ The kidneys may be unable to handle the task of getting rid of these by-products and may become damaged. ■ Damage to the kidneys usually develops gradually, and there are usually no signs of it. ■ Damage to the bladder happens quickly, with symptoms such as pain on urination or the passing of blood in the urine. ■ These symptoms are also a sign of a urinary tract infection. ■ If your child has any of these symptoms, tell his doctor immediately.

Damage to the kidneys or bladder may be permanent, so the kidneys and urine are checked frequently. ■ Fortunately, there are many simple and effective measures that can help prevent damage to the kidneys or bladder. ■ For instance, encouraging your child to empty his bladder often will reduce the time that harmful substances stay in his bladder. ■ Ask your child's doctor if this is necessary. ■ Sometimes, extra medications are given with, or before, your child's chemotherapy, which can prevent damage to the kidneys and bladder.

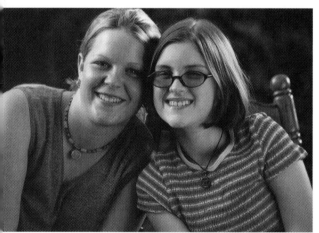

Reproductive System

Many anti-cancer drugs can affect the reproductive organs (ovaries, testicles). ■ We don't know how infants and very young children are affected. ■ In older children and adolescents, puberty may be delayed. ■ Adolescent girls may begin menstruation (periods) later or have irregular periods during treatment and afterwards. In a few cases, a young girl's ovaries may fail. ■ Her periods will stop, and menopausal symptoms will begin. ■ In adolescent boys, sperm production may be affected or eliminated. ■ These patients may wish to consider putting sperm in a sperm bank before beginning treatment. ■ Remember, while reduced fertility is a common side effect of chemotherapy, conception may still occur later in life.

Metabolism

While anti-cancer drugs have little effect on overall growth in children, they can have temporary effects on the body. ■ Minerals may be lost from bones, causing aches and pains in the bones and joints and possibly a limp while walking. ■ If too many minerals are lost, bone fractures may happen.

Some drugs will affect how the body breaks down and makes sugar, possibly causing a temporary diabetic state. ■ Your child may feel thirstier and urinate more often. ■ Other drugs may upset the body's salt and water balance, and your child may urinate less often. ■ If you notice these types of symptoms, tell your child's doctor immediately.

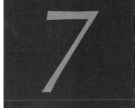

Many anti-cancer drugs can damage the liver. ■ In most cases, this damage is mild. ■ However, if the damage is repeated, the condition of the liver may grow worse over time. Your child will have his liver function measured regularly throughout therapy to watch for any signs of liver damage. ■ If damage is present and gets worse, the doses of certain medications may need to be changed.

Heart and Lungs

Certain anti-cancer drugs can damage the heart or lungs. ■ This damage usually happens slowly and grows each time the drug is given. ■ Your child will have regular testing of his heart and lungs if one of these drugs is needed for his treatment. This testing helps identify problems at an early stage, allowing the drug's dose to be changed. ■ Symptoms of heart or lung damage include discomfort in the chest, shortness of breath, and long-standing cough. ■ Tell your child's doctor if you notice any of these symptoms.

Immunity

Most anti-cancer drugs will affect your child's immune system, putting him at risk for developing infection. ■ Certain childhood illnesses such as chicken pox can be quite serious in your child. ■ Tell the clinic immediately if your child is exposed to another child who has, or develops, an illness like chicken pox. ■ It is generally safe for children on chemotherapy to continue receiving most of their usual immunizations on

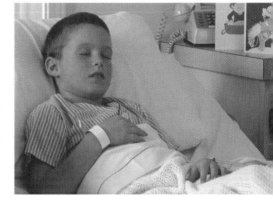

schedule. ■ But be sure to speak to your child's doctor before your child receives any vaccine.

Right Atrial Catheters

When intensive chemotherapy is given through a vein (intravenously), children can experience physical and emotional injury from frequent needle pokes. ■ When the same veins (usually in the arms) are used for an extended period of time, inflammation, blood clotting, or drug leakage from the vein into the skin may occur. ■ This can cause pain as well.

To avoid these problems, a right atrial catheter is commonly used. ■ This catheter is a narrow, flexible, sterile tube that allows easy access to veins. ■ It is placed in a large vein in the neck, with the tip in the smaller chamber (atrium) of the right side of the heart. ■ This is done usually under general anesthesia by a surgeon, who leads the other end of the tube from the neck vein through a tunnel under the skin to a distant point on the front of the chest. ■ The tunnel protects against infection and anchors the catheter so that it won't dislodge.

Right atrial catheters are a convenient way to take blood samples. ■ They also provide a route for giving
- anti-cancer drugs, antibiotics, and other medications
- blood products including red blood cells and platelets and other intravenous fluids
- total parenteral nutrition (see Chapter 13).

These catheters mean less time spent in the clinic, less emotional upset for children, parents, and staff, and less anticipatory vomiting (which can occur when a child is expecting an intravenous needle).

Two types of right atrial catheters are available. ■ The first type, called a Hickman™ or Broviac™ catheter, is partly external and lies several inches outside the exit site on the front of the chest. ■ It has a cap at the end and may have plastic clasps on the tubing itself to ensure that it is closed off when not in use. ■ The catheter must be flushed with a sterile solution and the covering sterile dressing changed regularly. ■ Breaks in the external tubing can be repaired. ■ The clinic staff can show you how to flush the catheter and change the dressing at home. ■ Repairs to the catheter, however, will have to be done by the staff. ■ Hickman or Broviac catheters are available in several sizes and as single and double tubes.

Another type of catheter, a Port-A-Cath™ (often called a "Port"), is an internal line placed completely under the skin. ■ This allows your child to participate in physical activities such as swimming. ■ Contact sports, however, are still not a good idea. ■ No dressings are required, and flushing is needed only once a month when the catheter is not in use.

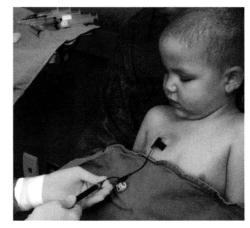

Special needles (called Huber needles) are needed to penetrate the skin and puncture the rubber seal to access internal catheters. ■ Fortunately, this procedure is much more comfortable now with the use of EMLA™ cream. ■ EMLA is applied to the Port site one to three hours before the procedure and numbs the area so that your child will not feel the needle. ■ EMLA may come as a cream secured with a transparent dressing or a patch that fits securely over the Port site.

Port-A-Caths are available in different sizes. ■ They may not be suitable for the (small) infant, although they may be used in children as young as two years of age.

Surface skin infections and serious blood-borne infections are less frequent with internal catheters, but they are not without problems:
• The skin overlying the Port site remains sensitive.
• Withdrawing blood samples can be more difficult than with external catheters.
• Blockages can occur.
• Rupture of the tubing within the chest wall can't be repaired.
• Although it doesn't happen often, anti-cancer drugs can leak and may cause a serious injury.

Despite these possible complications, both external and internal right atrial catheters are highly beneficial for the physical and emotional well-being of children having cancer treatment.

SURGERY IS AN IMPORTANT PART OF CANCER TREATMENT FOR CHILDREN. OFTEN, CHILDREN WITH CANCER NEED A SPECIAL CATHETER PLACED IN A LARGE VEIN (SEE CHAPTER 9—RIGHT ATRIAL CATHETERS). THIS CATHETER MAKES IT EASIER TO GIVE TREATMENT OR DRAW BLOOD.

An operation is often needed to determine the exact nature of the tumor (biopsy) and the extent of its spread (staging). ■ In some cases, all or most of the cancer can be removed. ■ In others, it is best to only biopsy the tumor and start treatment with chemotherapy and/or radiotherapy. ■ Sometimes, an operation is done following other treatments to see if any cancer remains. ■ This is called a "second-look" procedure. ■ Sometimes, surgery can relieve upsetting symptoms, even though cure may not be possible. ■ This is called a palliative operation.

The child, parent, and surgeon must work together to make sure the operation and recovery go as smoothly as possible. ■ You and your child may be frightened about an operation. ■ Don't hesitate to ask questions; writing them down as they come to mind helps. ■ You will be given open and honest answers. ■ Your surgeon is the best person to explain any details about the surgery.

The following are commonly asked questions and their answers. If other questions come to mind or you don't understand the answers, write the questions down and ask your surgeon.

Why is an operation needed? ■ An operation will be recommended only when the treatment team agrees that it is the best and safest method to find out the exact nature of the tumor, to attempt to remove it, to learn how far it has spread, or to insert a right atrial catheter.

Why are so many tests needed before the operation? ■ Laboratory and x-ray tests can help the surgeon get ready for the operation and ensure that it is as safe as it can be. ■ You will be told about each test and what is involved.

When will the operation take place? ■ We understand that you're anxious for the operation to take place. ■ However, it's important that all of the necessary tests and preparations be done first. ■ As soon as the exact time of the surgery is decided, you will be told so that you and your child can get ready. ■ Sometimes, the operation will be done outside the regular operating hours

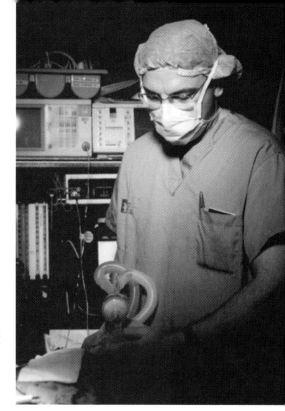

(on the "wait list"). ■ In this situation, you will be told an approximate time for the surgery. It is possible that the time will change if an emergency operation needs to be performed on another patient. ■ We will try to keep you as informed as possible.

How can you prepare your child? The best way to prepare your child is to be sure that you understand what is expected. ■ Then, explain everything openly to your child in a way he can understand. ■ Your honesty, understanding, and support will reassure him, and the child life staff, through explanation and play, can help your child feel less confused and afraid.

What sort of anesthetic will be used? Your child will be asleep and entirely unaware of what is going on during the operation (general anesthesia). ■ The anesthetist/anesthesiologist (the doctor who gives your child the anesthesia and watches him throughout the surgery) will visit before the operation to check your child carefully and will be happy to answer any of your questions.

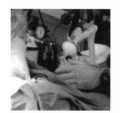

May I be with my child in the operating room? Some hospitals allow parents, along with a specially trained volunteer, to go with their child into the operating room while he is "going to sleep" under the anesthetic. ■ Your presence can be a great comfort to your child, but, at all times, his safety comes first. ■ Parents are generally allowed in the operating room for only low-risk, simple operations. They must have been oriented to the operating room already, and there must be a volunteer or extra nurse with them. ■ Please feel free to discuss this with your surgeon and anesthetist/anesthesiologist.

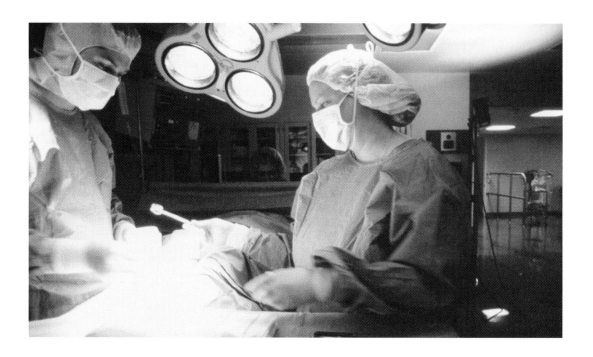

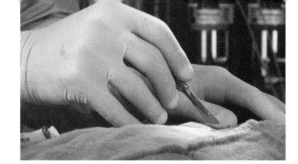

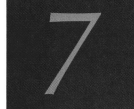

How risky is the anesthetic and the operation? With careful preparation, the risks will be reduced to an absolute minimum. ■ Some operations for cancer are difficult, but the risks must be balanced against the better chance of a cure. ■ Your surgeon and anesthetist will be open and honest with you about the risks and benefits of the surgery.

How long will the operation last? There are many steps that must occur in the operating room, so the length of the operation varies a great deal. ■ We can usually predict when it will finish, but don't be alarmed if the operation takes longer. ■ The surgeon always works carefully and never allows himself/herself to be rushed.

Where can we wait during the operation? You are encouraged to wait in the operating room waiting area, where you can be close to your child. ■ Your surgeon will meet you there after the operation is over. ■ If you wish to leave for a period of time during the operation, be sure to tell the receptionist where you can be reached, in case the operation finishes earlier than expected.

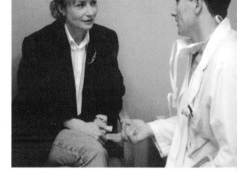

When will we be told the results of the surgery? When the operation is finished, your surgeon will tell you how the operation went. ■ If the operation lasts a long time, the surgeon will send out a nurse to give you information while it's going on. ■ If tissue was removed for examination under the microscope, it will be several days before the report is available. ■ Only then will we know the exact nature of the tumor. ■ The type of tumor will determine what other treatment is needed. ■ When this information is available, your child's doctor will talk to you about further treatment.

Where will my child be cared for after the surgery? Your child will be watched closely in the recovery room for a period of time after surgery. ■ You will be able to see your child in the recovery room once he is awake. ■ Then, your child will be moved back to the nursing care area; this could be the intensive care unit, intermediate care unit, pediatric surgery unit, or general pediatric ward. ■ Usually, the decision of where your child will be cared for is made before the operation. ■ But if the needs of your child change after surgery, he will be moved to the unit best suited to his care.

Will my child have pain after surgery? Your child will be sore after surgery, especially when he moves, breathes deeply, or coughs. ■ With your help, we can reduce pain as much as possible. ■ It's a good idea for your child to move, cough, and breathe deeply to help prevent complications and speed recovery. ■ Pain medication can be given as needed but more commonly is given continuously through a vein. ■ If your child is old enough, he may be taught before the surgery about a special machine (PCA pump) that allows him to give himself extra pain medication (up to a limit). ■ This can be discussed with your child's surgeon, nurse, anesthetist/anesthesiologist, or pain specialist.

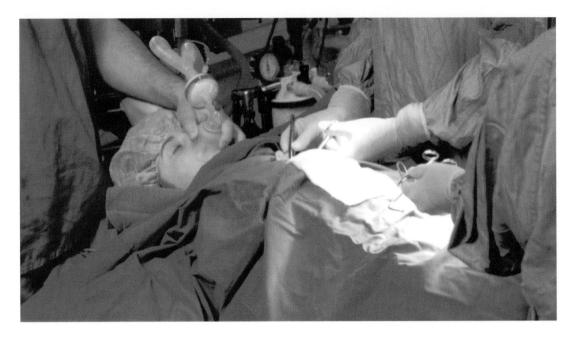

Why does my child need all of those wires and tubes? If your child is in the intensive or intermediate care unit, his pulse rate, temperature, and blood pressure may be visible on monitors that look like television screens. ■ This can be frightening if you don't understand what is happening, so be sure to ask. ■ Usually, fluids will be given through an intravenous line to avoid thirst and to allow medication to be given without many injections. ■ Sometimes, the doctor needs to measure the exact amount of urine that your child is able to produce. If so, a small tube (catheter) is left in the bladder.

What are those other tubes? Vomiting and gas pains, often resulting from an abdominal operation, can be avoided with a nasogastric tube to keep the stomach empty. ■ This is a small tube passed from the nose into the stomach. ■ After a chest operation, a chest tube may be left in place to help the lung expand properly. ■ Sometimes, a wound drain is left to allow unwanted fluids to escape. ■ All of these devices are removed easily as soon as they have done their jobs.

What complications may occur? Fortunately, complications after surgery are less common in children than in adults. ■ Sometimes, after the operation, internal bleeding occurs, and a transfusion is needed. ■ Only in a very few cases, a second operation is done to control the bleeding. ■ Breathing problems may develop if your child doesn't want to breathe deeply and cough; this is one reason pain control is so important. ■ If necessary, the physiotherapist will help your child with breathing exercises. ■ Sometimes, children have problems urinating, and a bladder catheter is put in. Even with the right steps, poor healing or wound infection can occur, so extra treatment, like antibiotics, may be needed. ■ Please be sure to ask the surgeon about any other risks related to your child's surgery.

Will there be a big, ugly scar? Every surgical operation leaves a scar, but your child's surgeon will try to leave a scar that is the least noticeable it can be. ■ The appearance of the scar will continue to improve for a full year after the operation.

L IKE CHEMOTHERAPY, RADIATION ATTACKS CANCER CELLS AND THEIR ABILITY TO GROW AND DIVIDE. RADIATION THERAPY IS SOMETIMES CALLED "RADIOTHERAPY," "X-RAY THERAPY," OR "IRRADIATION."

Uses of Radiation Therapy

R adiation can be used to treat cancers in almost every part of the body and is usually focused to treat just the area of the cancer. ■ Radiation therapy can be given as a treatment alone or in combination with surgery and chemotherapy. ■ Treatment is aimed at curing the cancer or relieving symptoms. ■ It can also be used to prevent the spread of cancer (such as leukemia) to other parts of the body.

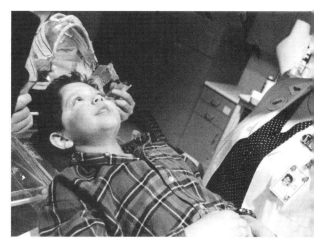

Deciding on Treatment Dose

T he amount or dose of radiation needed to cure a specific tumor is known from past experience around the world. ■ Some tumors are more sensitive to radiation than others, and larger tumors may need more radiation than smaller ones. ■ The dose will depend on how much radiation the normal cells can take. ■ Some anti-cancer drugs make tumor cells and normal tissues more sensitive to radiation, so the dose of radiation will have to be changed in children receiving these drugs. ■ Often, changes to dose are made in very young children. ■ Many things affect the timing and dose of radiation for a child. ■ Some children will need more treatments over a longer period than other children; this does not mean that their cancer is more serious.

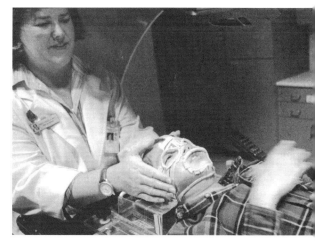

Where and How Radiation Therapy Is Given

T he treatment is given in the radiation therapy department. ■ The radiation oncologist and liaison nurse (if there is one) will meet with your family at the hospital when radiation is used to treat your child. ■ At this time, they will examine him and discuss the treatment in detail. ■ They will also give you written information about radiation therapy, how long the treatment will last, and possible side effects. You are encouraged to ask questions. ■ The child life staff will help explain the treatment to your child in terms he will understand.

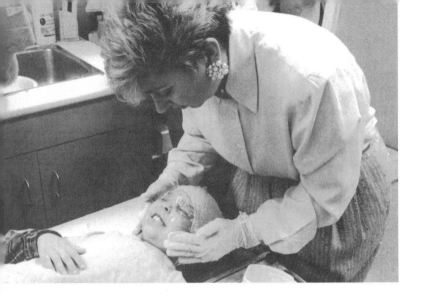

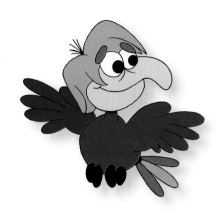

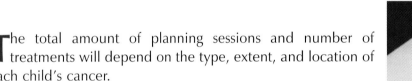

Planning Radiation Therapy

To work well, radiation therapy must be planned carefully before actually starting the treatment. ■ This planning often takes place in two stages:

The making of a mold:	**Stage 1**
Simulation:	**Stage 2**

The total amount of planning sessions and number of treatments will depend on the type, extent, and location of each child's cancer.

During the first stage, a plastic mold will often be made of the area to receive radiation. ■ This light-weight plastic cast will help your child to stay in the same position during each planning and treatment time. ■ Marks will be drawn on the cast in the next phase. ■ Very young children may need sedation so that they can hold still for the planning and treatments.

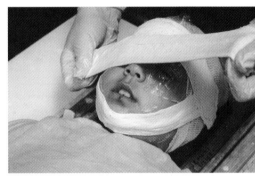

The second stage of planning is called simulation. ■ Your child will be asked to lie very still on a table while a radiation therapist uses an x-ray machine (called a simulator or CAT simulator) to find the exact place on the body where the treatment will be aimed. ■ The therapist will mark on the plastic shell the area that will be treated. ■ Plain x-rays or CAT scans may be taken. ■ Simulation may take several appointments, each appointment lasting up to one hour. ■ You or another family member can usually be present.

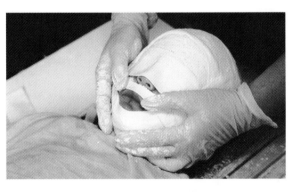

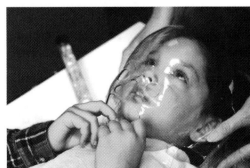

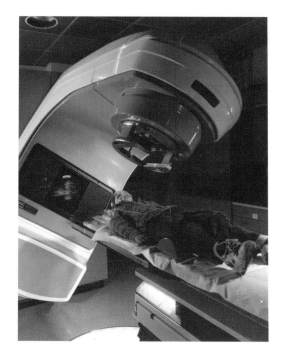

Radiation Treatment

There is no pain in the planning stages or treatment. ■ The number of treatments needed varies; often, as many as 30 treatments are needed. ■ You will be given a daily schedule of the treatment times. ■ In the treatment room, your child is positioned, and the mold is put on the area to receive treatment. ■ Time is spent making sure the marks on the cast line up with the machine settings. ■ Your child must remain still.

Once the therapists have checked the position of your child, the marks on the cast, and the treatment machine settings, they will leave the treatment room. ■ Your child is secured for safety. ■ He can be seen on a TV and heard through a speaker. ■ You and the radiation therapist can talk to your child during this time to provide encouragement and support. ■ Your child is alone in the treatment room only for a minute or two during treatment and is watched constantly. ■ He is able to talk to you and the staff, unless heavily sedated.

The treatment machines are large and make noise as they move around to aim the treatment from different angles. ■ The machine never touches your child and he can't see, hear, or feel the radiation. ■ Each treatment appointment will last between 10 minutes and a half hour.

Common Side Effects of Treatment

When treating cancer, normal cells can be affected. ■ Side effects depend on the area of the body treated and the number of treatments given. ■ If the head, or part of it, is treated, your child may lose hair in this area, sometimes permanently, depending on the amount of radiation given. ■ If large areas of the body are treated, nausea and vomiting may occur, although they can usually be completely prevented by medication. ■ Your child may be more tired than usual during the period of treatment, but this wears off once the treatment is finished.

The radiation oncologist will watch for these side effects and will examine your child often. ■ The possible side effects, both short and long term, will be discussed with you and your child at the first visit. ■ You will be given written materials and instructions about managing any side effects from radiation treatment.

CHAPTER 7 IN BRIEF

Chemotherapy

Chemotherapy means treatment with medication (chemicals). Given by mouth or injection, drugs travel through the bloodstream, attacking and killing cancer cells in your child's body. At the same time, however, your child's muscles, nerves, urinary tract, reproductive organs, heart, lungs, and overall immunity may be injured. During treatment, your child may experience hair loss, fatigue, pain in his arms and legs, and sores in his mouth. Most of these side effects are temporary and improve with adjustments to the medication. Effective drugs are now available to prevent and treat nausea and vomiting commonly associated with chemotherapy.

Surgery

There are many different reasons for your child to have surgery. The type of cancer and the size and site of the tumor will help decide if an operation is needed. Your child will not have an operation unless we believe it is the best option. Risks related to surgery are kept to an absolute minimum. Happily, as compared to adults, complications after surgery are less frequent and the recovery time much shorter for children. To help speed recovery and manage any pain, the nurse and physiotherapist may give your child exercises to do. Encourage your child to cooperate.

Radiation Therapy

Radiation therapy is another way to kill some cancer cells and may be given along with chemotherapy and surgery. Radiation has no sound and is invisible, and the machine never touches your child. Treatment only lasts a few minutes; during this time, you may talk to your child through a microphone and watch him on a TV screen. Radiation therapy may have some unpleasant, but usually temporary, side effects such as hair loss, nausea, vomiting, fatigue, and skin changes. There may be some long-term effects that your child's radiation oncologist and nurse can tell you about.

NOTES

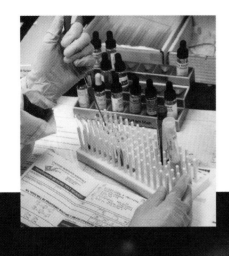

HEMORRHAGE AND THROMBOSIS

CHILDREN WITH CANCER MAY HAVE UNUSUAL BLEEDING (HEMORRHAGE) OR CLOTTING (THROMBOSIS) FOR MANY DIFFERENT REASONS.

The following discussion will explain normal blood clotting (hemostasis), the problems that can develop with blood clotting in children with cancer, and the diagnosis and treatment of these problems.

Normal Hemostasis

In the body, there is a fine balance between blood clotting and bleeding. ■ This normal situation is maintained by three different things:

1. Blood vessels

Blood vessels help stop bleeding by narrowing (contracting).

2. Platelets

When there is damage to a blood vessel, blood cells called platelets stick to the blood vessel wall and release chemicals that bring other platelets to the damaged area.

3. Proteins

There are also proteins that help form a blood clot. ■ These proteins react with each other in a domino effect. ■ The first protein becomes active when damage to a blood vessel occurs. ■ This protein then activates the second protein, which then activates the third protein, and so on until the final protein becomes active. ■ This final protein forms a strong material that, together with platelets, forms the blood clot at the site of the injury. ■ There are also proteins that thin the blood, which prevents too much blood clotting.

Cancer and its treatment can create problems with any of these three things, resulting in an unusual increase in bleeding or clotting.

Hemorrhage

Different types of chemotherapy and radiation not only kill the cancer cells but also normal cells, which produce platelets. ■ If the number of platelets gets too low, there is a greater risk of bleeding (hemorrhage).

Many patients with cancer eat poorly and don't get enough vitamins. Vitamin K, for instance, is needed to produce some of the proteins needed for blood clotting. ■ If a child doesn't get enough vitamin K, he may have abnormal bleeding (hemorrhage).

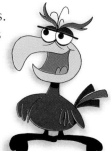

Many blood clotting proteins are produced by the liver. ■ Some cancers and their treatment can damage the liver. ■ If there's enough damage, there aren't enough clotting proteins for normal blood clotting.

In a few patients with cancer, proteins are produced that stop the clotting of blood, which may lead to hemorrhage.

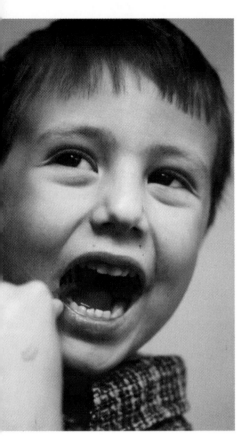

Signs of Hemorrhage

There are many signs that tell if a patient is bleeding (hemorrhaging) or may be at risk for bleeding. ■ If you notice any of the following signs, immediately contact your child's doctor or nurse:

- Bleeding when brushing the teeth
- Blood in the urine (hematuria)
- Blood in the stool (hematochezia)—fresh blood or black, tarry stools
- Vomiting of blood (hematemesis)—fresh blood or "coffee-ground" vomit
- Coughing up blood (hemoptysis)
- Severe nosebleeds (epistaxis)
- Severe bleeding following a cut or other injury
- A pin-point red-purple rash on the skin or inside the mouth (petechiae)
- Large bruises that can't be explained (ecchymoses)
- Severe headache that won't go away
- A fit (seizure)
- Unusual behavior that isn't explained by any other cause

Diagnosing Hemorrhage

The reason for a hemorrhage can be discovered by doing a complete blood count to measure the platelet count and other tests to tell how well the clotting system is working. ■ Sometimes, special tests are needed to take a closer look.

Treating Hemorrhage

In most cases, a patient with a hemorrhage can be treated. ■ If the platelet count is far too low, an injection of platelets (transfusion) can be given. ■ If bleeding is due to a decrease in the amount, or the activity of, the clotting proteins, then plasma or purified protein concentrate can be given through a vein (intravenously). ■ If a child isn't getting enough vitamin K, then more can be given.

Thrombosis

Cancer and its treatment can interfere with the production of proteins that stop clotting naturally. ■ If this occurs, blood flow slows, and a blood clot can form (thrombosis). ■ A blood clot is a clump that results when blood changes from liquid to solid (coagulates). ■ A blood clot in a deep vein can partially or completely stop the flow of blood. ■ It can also break off and travel through the bloodstream to the lungs, brain, heart, or any other area, where it can cause severe damage and even death.

Right atrial catheters (see Chapter 7) may increase the chance of blood clots forming in the large veins in the upper body. ■ Some of these clots may move to the lungs (pulmonary emboli), and this can be a serious, sometimes life-threatening, problem.

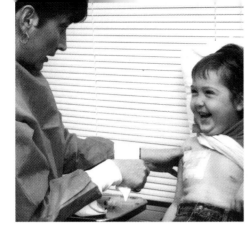

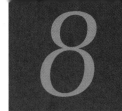

Signs of Thrombosis

There are many signs of a blood clot. ■ If you notice any of the following signs, immediately contact your child's doctor or nurse:

- Swelling and pain in an arm or leg
- Swelling and/or pain in the neck or face if a right atrial catheter is in place
- Inability to flush a right atrial catheter
- Dilated blood vessels on the neck or side of the face

The following signs could mean there is a blood clot in the lungs (pulmonary embolus):

- Sudden shortness of breath
- Chest pain
- Blueness of nail beds or lips

The following signs could mean there is a blood clot in the brain (stroke):

- Severe headache
- Nausea and/or vomiting
- Seizures that can't be explained
- Uncontrolled shaking of an arm or leg
- Loss of consciousness
- Drooping of one side of the mouth or face
- Unexplained weakness of an arm or leg

Diagnosing Thrombosis

Blood clots in the arms or legs or a large central blood vessel are diagnosed usually with a test called a venogram. ■ This test involves injecting a special dye into the vein and taking x-rays to see if the vein is blocked. ■ If the test can't be done, an ultrasound of the vein is carried out. ■ This method may not be as good at finding blood clots, and some of them may be missed.

Blood clots in the lungs are diagnosed with a special test called a lung scan. ■ A small amount of a radioactive material is injected into a vein, and another is inhaled. ■ Scans of the images from the blood vessels in the lungs and from the air sacs are compared to see if a blood clot is present. ■ Rarely, a special test called a pulmonary angiogram is needed to diagnose a blood clot in the lungs. ■ With this test, dye is injected into the large blood vessel (the pulmonary artery) that supplies the lungs.

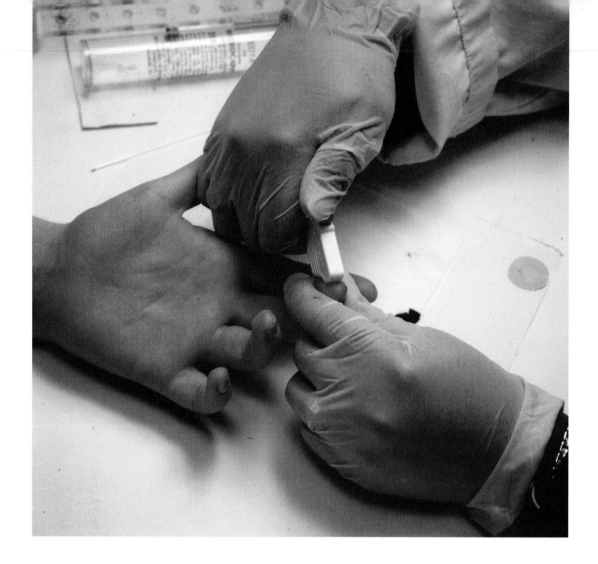

Blood clots in the brain are diagnosed with either a special technique called magnetic resonance imaging (MRI) or by injecting dye into the blood vessels of the brain (cerebral angiogram).

Treating Thrombosis
• Blood clot in the arm or leg or large blood vessel in the upper or lower body

Blood thinners (anticoagulants), called heparin and coumadin, are given either intravenously or under the skin (subcutaneously) in the case of heparin or by mouth (orally) in the case of coumadin. ■ Your child will be watched closely to make sure there is the right amount of drug in the blood.

Getting blood samples from children can be difficult, although a home blood monitor, which uses a finger poke to get blood, may be used.

In certain cases, for example, clots caused by right atrial catheters, treatment to help break up the clot is given (lytic therapy). ■ The drugs are given intravenously for a few minutes to several hours. ■ Blood thinners are also given at the same time, and then for some time afterwards. ■ In many cases, the right atrial catheter must be removed.

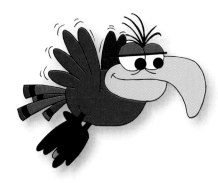

• **Blood clot in the lung**

At first, some children will be treated with drugs to help break up the clot. ■ Then, a blood thinner will usually be given. ■ Some children will also need oxygen therapy and pain medications.

• **Blood clot in the brain**

Patients with certain types of brain clots are treated with blood thinners if there's no bleeding into the brain itself.

CHAPTER 8 IN BRIEF

In children with cancer, the normal blood clotting process may not work properly, due either to the cancer itself or its treatment. Your child may experience more bleeding than is normal; this is called a hemorrhage. Or your child may develop the opposite problem of increased blood clotting; this is called thrombosis.

There are signs and symptoms that indicate if your child is experiencing a hemorrhage or thrombosis; a complete list is provided in this chapter. If you notice any one of them, speak to a nurse or doctor immediately. In most cases, the cause of a hemorrhage or thrombosis can be found through special tests and effective treatment given to your child.

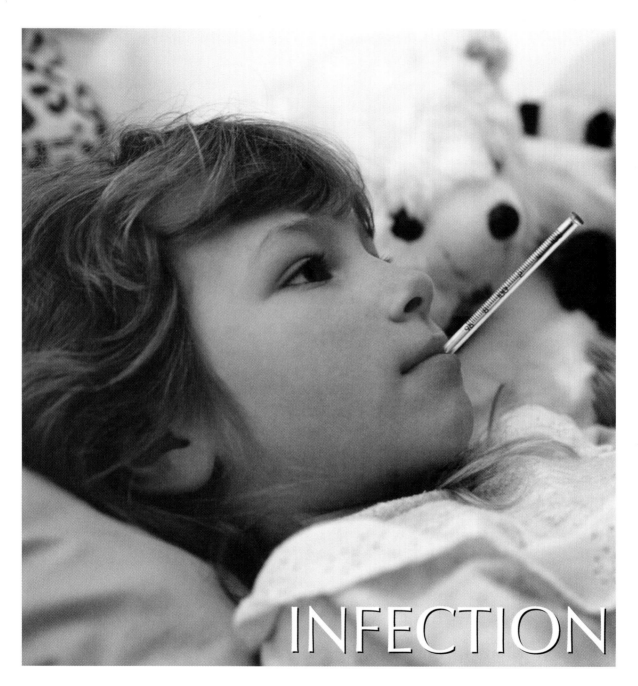

INFECTION
AND THE CHILD
WITH CANCER

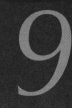
ONE OF THE MOST IMPORTANT PROBLEMS FACING CHILDREN WITH CANCER IS A GREATER CHANCE OF GETTING A SERIOUS INFECTION.

The cancer and its treatment, namely chemotherapy and radiation therapy, weaken the body's ability to defend itself from germs that cause infection. ■ The good news is that there are ways to prevent infections and successfully treat them with medicines if they do begin. ■ Since treatment works best in the early stages of infection, it's important for you to recognize the early signs of infection so that you can get medical advice as soon as possible.

Why do people on cancer treatment have problems with infections?

Body surfaces, such as the skin and the linings of the mouth and intestines, are important shields against germs, but when they're damaged, germs can invade the body. ■ This damage can be caused by surgery, accidental injury, repeated jabs for blood tests and intravenous injections, radiotherapy, and chemotherapy. ■ Radiotherapy occasionally burns the skin, and chemotherapy sometimes causes painful sores in the mouth where the lining has been damaged temporarily.

Neutrophils are white blood cells, produced in the bone marrow, that kill germs throughout the body. ■ Unfortunately, cancer treatments can temporarily stop the bone marrow from producing neutrophils so that the number falls too low and germs can invade.

Lymphocytes are another type of white blood cell that may be affected by cancer treatment. ■ Some chemotherapy reduces the number of lymphocytes for long periods, putting a child at risk of severe forms of chicken pox and of a particular type of lung infection caused by the germ known as *Pneumocystis carinii*. ■ Although chicken pox and *Pneumocystis carinii* lung infections in children with cancer can be treated, there are simple ways to prevent them in the first place.

What can be done to prevent infection in children with cancer?

Whenever possible, children with cancer should not be around other people who might have serious infections. ■ While in hospital, children with cancer are kept in protected areas so that the germs of the other patients do not reach them. ■ When your child's neutrophil count is very low, he should stay away from public places (schools, malls, movie theatres) where there might be people carrying harmful germs. ■ When neutrophil counts are not low, your child should enjoy life as much as possible without fear of germs from other people. ■ If a family member is ill, ask your child's doctor if special precautions are needed.

If your child has a right atrial catheter (such as a Hickman or Port-A-Cath), take special care that the line doesn't become infected. ■ Try to follow the instructions given by your child's

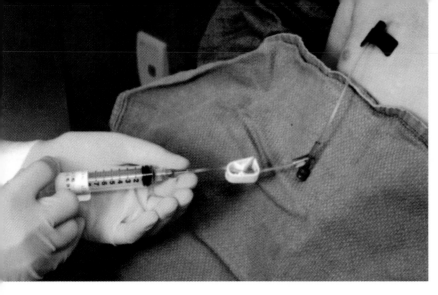

doctors and nurses who help take care of these lines. ■ If the area around the line becomes red or sore or shows a discharge of fluid, call the doctor immediately.

If your child has never had chicken pox, he may get a severe form of it after being around another child who is in the early stages of the infection. ■ If you think your child was exposed to a case of chicken pox, contact your child's doctor immediately. ■ Chicken pox can be prevented with an early injection of antibodies directed against the chicken pox virus. ■ These specially prepared antibodies, called varicella-zoster immune globulin (VZIG), are taken from healthy blood donors (see Chapter 10). ■ If your child did have chicken pox before he developed cancer, it's not likely he will get chicken pox again. ■ In this case, special precautions and injections of VZIG are usually not needed.

Cold sores are caused by a virus known as herpes simplex. ■ This virus can be spread by kissing while cold sores can be seen on the lip of the affected person. ■ Anyone with cold sores should stay away from children with cancer. ■ Hand washing and automatic dishwashers are good ways of stopping the spread of herpes simplex virus from one person to another in a household.

If your child is being given treatment that increases his chances of getting *Pneumocystis carinii* infection of the lungs, the doctors will give him medicine to prevent that infection. ■ This medicine is given orally or sometimes intravenously. ■ He will take this medicine for months or even years—one or two doses per day, three days per week.

What are the signs of infection that families should look for?

Fever over 38°C/100°F means that your child probably has an infection. ■ In children with cancer, it can be difficult to know if the infection is mild or serious. ■ If the neutrophil count is low at the time of fever, there is a chance that there could be bacteria in the bloodstream. ■ Infections of the bloodstream must be treated with intravenous antibiotics immediately. ■ Keep a reliable thermometer handy and learn how to take the temperature either by mouth or under the armpit. ■ If your child has a fever, call the doctor or nurse right away.

Redness, tenderness, or discharge at the site of an intravenous line means that the line is probably infected. ■ Call the doctor immediately so your child can receive the proper treatment before the infection gets worse or complications develop.

Spots on the skin that look like small blisters may be the first sign of chicken pox. ■ Chicken pox can be treated successfully with intravenous medicine such as acyclovir. But acyclovir only works well if it is given within a day or two after the spots first appear. ■ Delays in treating chicken pox in some children with cancer can be life-threatening. ■ If you think your child has chicken pox, call the doctor on the same day you first see the spots. ■ DO NOT go to the clinic, as your child may pass on the infection to others. ■ You will be told over the phone about bringing your child to the hospital/clinic.

A rash on the skin may be the first sign of infection. ■ If you see a rash and don't know what it is, call the doctor or nurse.

A cough may be due to a simple virus infection or to a serious lung infection such as *Pneumocystis carinii*. ■ If your child develops a cough that lasts more than a day, call the doctor. ■ The doctor will examine your child and may wish to order a chest x-ray to find out the reason for the cough.

How are infections treated?
Serious bacterial infections are treated with combinations of antibiotics, given intravenously for a week or two. ■ To find out the exact nature of the infection, the doctors will order tests such as blood work, x-rays, and ultrasounds. ■ Some tests are uncomfortable, but they are necessary to diagnose and treat serious infections.

Sometimes, a fever doesn't come down even after several days of treatment. ■ One reason may be that the neutrophil count stays so low that the medicine can't get rid of the germs or because other germs called fungi have come along. ■ Fungi can be treated with a special medication (such as amphotericin B), although many children have chills, shivers, and nausea when they take it. ■ Other medicines can help relieve these uncomfortable side effects. ■ The younger the child, the milder the side effects.

Pneumocystis carinii lung infections are treated with high doses of medicine, given orally or intravenously.

Do children with cancer have regular vaccinations (immunization)?
Children who are being treated for cancer should not be given live virus vaccines such as measles, rubella, mumps, and oral polio. ■ These vaccines are usually given at least three months after treatment has finished. ■ However, there are certain vaccines that can be given during cancer treatment, including

- diluted Hib
- Pneumovax
- influenza.

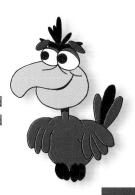

Your child's doctor can tell you when it is safe and necessary for your child to have any vaccinations. ■ Be sure to tell the doctor if he has received previous vaccinations.

CHAPTER 9 IN BRIEF

Cancer and cancer treatments can make your child more susceptible to infection. Body surfaces, like the skin and lining of the mouth, may lose their ability to protect your child from infection, and his immune system may not work properly.

Infections in children with cancer can be severe, so learn to recognize when your child is at risk. Practice prevention, and if your child is exposed to chicken pox, inform your child's doctor as soon as possible. Most of all, help your child to practice good personal hygiene, such as regular hand washing. The greatest risk of infection is from his own normal bacteria found in his stools and on his skin.

There are different rules for giving vaccinations to children with cancer. Your child's doctor will give you a schedule designed to suit your child's needs. Vaccinations are usually provided by a family physician or pediatrician who will need to know your child's blood counts before giving the "shot."

While it's vital to protect your child from infection, so too is encouraging a normal, active life. Try to find a healthy balance. If your child does develop an infection, there are effective treatments such as antibiotics and drugs that fight viruses. Your child may need to stay in the hospital for a short time to receive these medications.

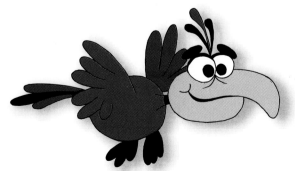

NOTES

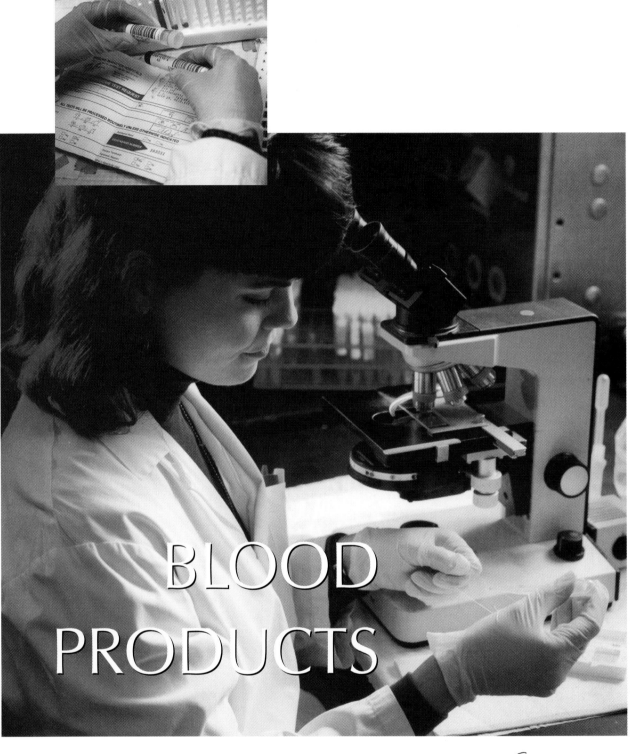

BLOOD PRODUCTS

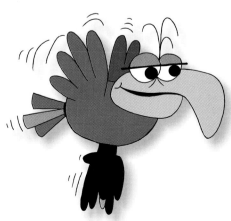

FROM TIME TO TIME, YOUR CHILD MAY NEED AN INJECTION OF BLOOD (TRANSFUSION)—USUALLY RED BLOOD CELLS, PLATELETS, OR PLASMA PRODUCTS.

Plasma is the straw-colored part of the blood. ■ Red blood cells may be given when your child's red blood cell levels are too low (anemia). ■ When his platelet count is low, he may bleed and bruise more easily. ■ When this happens, platelet transfusions may be given. Plasma products can be given to increase certain proteins in your child's blood.

Blood Typing and Crossmatching

Before blood is transfused, a sample of your child's blood is taken and tested to find out his blood type—A, B, AB, or O—and whether he is Rhesus positive or negative. ■ A special identification number, along with your child's name and hospital number, is placed on the blood sample. ■ Your child is then given an armband to wear. ■ The same three pieces of information are on the armband.

In the laboratory, another test mixes your child's blood with some of the red cells from blood from a donor. ■ This is called crossmatching. ■ If the donor blood doesn't match (incompatible), the red cells will clump together (agglutination). ■ If the blood matches (compatible), no clumping is seen. ■ Only compatible blood is given to your child. ■ Some people produce new antibodies after a blood transfusion is given, so a specimen of blood must be taken from the child each time a blood transfusion is needed. ■ If new antibodies have been made, the laboratory will see them in the crossmatch, and only compatible blood will be chosen for transfusion.

Red Cell Transfusion

Red cells are often given when their level has fallen too low or when major surgery is needed. ■ Before a transfusion, two nurses will formally confirm that the blood given by the blood bank carries the same three pieces of identification on your child's armband. ■ This is done to make sure your child receives the right blood. ■ A transfusion usually takes two to four hours.

Platelet Transfusion

Often, platelets are given to prevent bleeding in a child who has a low platelet count (thrombocytopenia). ■ There are two ways to get platelets for transfusion:

1 They can be separated from the individual bags of blood collected at blood donor clinics. ■ These are called random donor platelets. ■ Several random donors are usually needed to give your child enough platelets to prevent bleeding.

2 Large numbers of platelets can be collected from one donor using a piece of equipment called a plateletpheresis machine. ■ Blood from the donor enters the machine. ■ It

removes the platelets and then gives the red cells back to the donor. ■ Platelets collected by this method are equal to platelets given by five or six random donors.

At first, most children receive random donor platelet transfusions. ■ However, after many transfusions, your child may develop antibodies that attack the random donor platelets. ■ The physician will know when this happens because the platelet count in your child's blood does not rise after the transfusion. ■ If this happens, the blood bank will give single donor platelets since they may survive better after transfusion and may be better at preventing bruising and bleeding.

Plasma Products for Transfusion

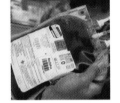

Children receiving chemotherapy have a greater chance of developing serious complications if they develop chicken pox. ■ If your child has been near someone who has chicken pox or shingles, he may be given a blood product called varicella-zoster immune globulin (VZIG). ■ VZIG is injected into the muscle within 72 hours of your child being exposed to chicken pox.

Transfusion of plasma may also be used to replace proteins that have been lowered by cancer and its treatment. ■ There is no need to do a crossmatch test before giving plasma.

Side Effects of Blood Transfusions

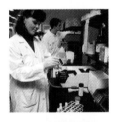

During blood transfusions, about five percent of people will have unpleasant side effects (transfusion reactions). ■ Side effects include chills, fevers and hives, wheezing, and tightness in the chest. ■ These symptoms usually appear within an hour of starting the transfusion but are usually temporary and only last for a few minutes to an hour. ■ Your child's vital signs will be watched during the transfusion. ■ Drugs, known as antihistamines, can control these reactions, so it is usually not necessary to stop the transfusion.

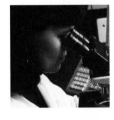

The laboratory will try to find out what caused this reaction in your child so it can be avoided next time. ■ For example, if the child develops a fever because of a reaction to the white cells in the donor blood, the blood bank can remove most of the white cells from the next donation and prevent another reaction from happening. ■ Your child may also be given antihistamines or Tylenol before the transfusion to prevent a reaction.

Some diseases can be spread by blood transfusions; hepatitis is the most common. ■ Be assured that all donors are carefully tested to prevent the spread of the most common viruses (B and C) that cause hepatitis. ■ Now, there are very few people who develop hepatitis from blood transfusions.

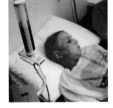

The virus that causes acquired immune deficiency syndrome (AIDS) is another virus that can be spread by transfusion. ■ All blood donors are screened for the AIDS virus, so the risk of getting AIDS from a transfusion is very rare (less than 1 in 200,000).

Reducing Side Effects from Blood Transfusions

It is now common practice to make changes to blood products before they are used to reduce the likelihood of viral infections and other side effects. ■ Below are two examples of how blood products are changed:

- Before transfusion, white blood cells (leukocytes) may be filtered out of products containing red blood cells and platelets. The end result is called a leukocyte-reduced cellular blood product.

- For children who have severely weakened immune systems (such as those who have recently had a bone marrow transplant), we often treat blood products with radiation before transfusion to reduce the risk of graft-versus-host disease (see Chapter 11).

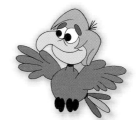

CHAPTER 10 IN BRIEF

From time to time, your child may require a transfusion (IV injection) of red blood cells or platelets. If your child is exposed to chicken pox, he may need to be treated with a blood product called VZIG. Be assured that every precaution is taken to guarantee that these blood products are safe. Screening procedures have significantly reduced the risk of contracting diseases like hepatitis or AIDS.

During a transfusion, your child may experience minor side effects like fever or hives. Antihistamines and acetaminophen (like Tylenol) can often prevent or control these types of reactions.

Blood products are an important way to safeguard the well-being of your child and maintain as normal a life as possible. These products are commonly altered to reduce the risk of side effects such as viral infections.

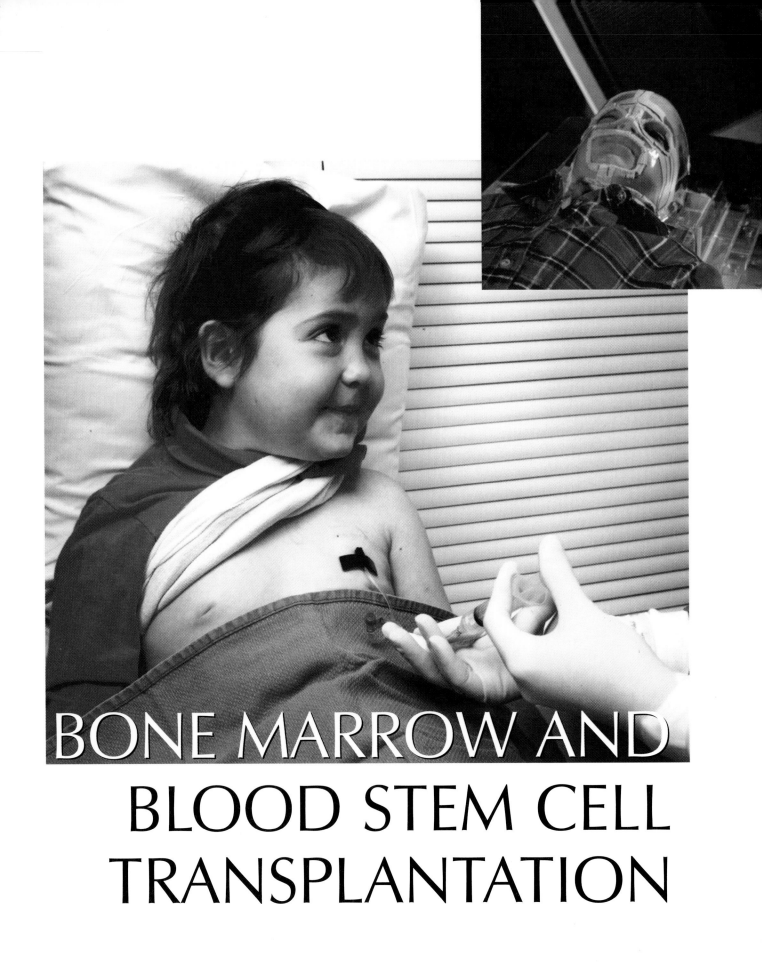

BONE MARROW AND BLOOD STEM CELL TRANSPLANTATION

THE BONE MARROW IS LOCATED IN THE CENTER OF MANY BONES IN THE BODY. IT IS THE PLACE WHERE MILLIONS OF CELLS ARE PRODUCED AND RELEASED INTO THE BLOODSTREAM EACH DAY.

Some of the cells produced in the bone marrow are called stem cells. ■ They are the origin of all of the other blood cells. ■ Some stem cells circulate in the blood.

Bone marrow is sensitive and can be injured by drugs (including chemotherapy) and by radiation. ■ Usually, this injury is temporary, and, as the bone marrow recovers, the child's blood counts return to normal. ■ Sometimes, the bone marrow is destroyed permanently, and the child needs a bone marrow transplantation.

Two types of bone marrow transplants (allogeneic and autologous) and blood stem cell transplants are being used more and more to treat childhood cancers and other blood disorders. ■ The type of transplant recommended by your child's doctor depends on the type of cancer and if a suitable donor is found.

Allogeneic Bone Marrow Transplant

Allo means "other." ■ Allogeneic bone marrow transplant uses cells donated by another person. ■ Because the cells come from another person, the immune system of the person receiving the cells (called the recipient) sees them as "foreign" cells and attacks them. ■ This immune response is a normal and important defense against infection, but it can also mean that transplanted bone marrow cells are destroyed. ■ This is called rejection.

To reduce the chance of rejection, the marrow to be transplanted (donor marrow) must be similar or matched to the recipient. ■ Children inherit genes from each parent, so parents are usually not suitable donors. ■ Brothers and sisters may have inherited the same set of genes from both parents and may be suitable donors. ■ A related donor, such as a brother or sister, is always best.

If no family members are suitable matches, an unrelated donor may be found through a Bone Marrow Registry, a listing of volunteers whose genetic type is known. ■ A computer compares the child's genetic type with the genetic type of all of the people in the registry in the hope of finding a match.

Once a match is found, your child will receive chemotherapy and/or radiation over several days in the hospital to get his body ready for the transplant. ■ First, the chemotherapy and/or radiation attacks any tumor or other "sick" cells that may still be present. ■ Second, it slows your child's immune system so that he will accept the donor's marrow. ■ This preparation is different for each child and depends on the cancer and the closeness of the match.

When this preparation is finished, the donor's marrow is transplanted into your child. ■ An operation isn't needed. Instead, the marrow is injected through a right atrial catheter (see Chapter 7), like a blood transfusion. ■ It's not painful. The marrow cells flow through the bloodstream and settle in the bone marrow.

Once this is done, the stem cells must settle in their new home and start producing new red blood cells, white blood cells, and platelets. ■ This is a slow process (called engraftment) and may take many days. ■ During this time, your child has a greater risk of infection, and many red cell and platelet transfusions are needed to avoid getting sick. ■ Your child may have a fever, diarrhea, and a sore mouth. ■ Special feeding (total parenteral nutrition or TPN – see Chapter 13) through the catheter is needed, and your child is placed in a room with special air filters to keep germs away.

When the blood counts have recovered and your child is eating well, he can leave hospital. ■ He will be watched carefully for six months or more since it may take many months before his immune system returns to normal.

Graft-Versus-Host Disease

Although the donor and recipient marrow are closely matched, they are almost never exactly the same, except with identical twins. ■ Once the donor's marrow has started producing new blood cells, it begins to recognize its new home as foreign and often tries to attack it. ■ This is called graft-versus-host disease. ■ This disease commonly affects the skin, liver, and gut. ■ The skin may become red or leathery, and jaundice and diarrhea also occur. ■ Fortunately, this disease can be controlled with medications such as cyclosporin and steroids. ■ Graft-versus-host disease has some good effects as well: it attacks any remaining cancer cells that may have survived the transplant. ■ Graft-versus-host disease is almost never seen in autologous transplants (see below).

Autologous Bone Marrow Transplant

Auto means "self." In an autologous bone marrow transplant, your child's own bone marrow is removed and then given back to him later. ■ First, he is taken to the operating room, and some of his bone marrow (usually less than a pint) is collected from his hip bone. ■ This is called the "harvest." The bone marrow that has been removed may be treated in a special way (called "purging") to remove any cancer cells. ■ Afterwards, there may be some bruising and soreness, but often your child can move around within a few hours. ■ He is then treated with several days of chemotherapy and/or radiation.

Once the chemotherapy and/or radiation is finished, the autologous bone marrow is injected back into your child. ■ The next steps are the same as those for allogeneic transplant (see above), except the preparation is usually less intense, and your child often recovers more quickly. ■ This is because he is receiving his own bone marrow.

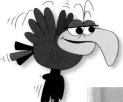

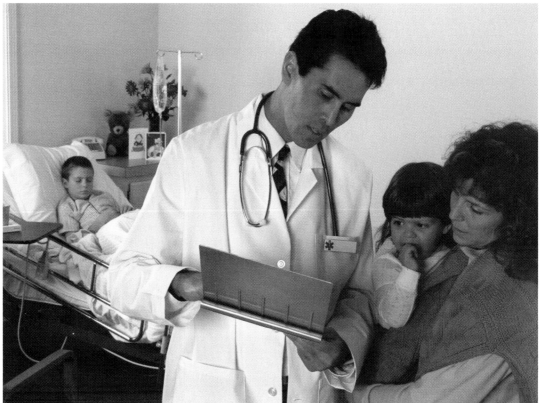

Peripheral Blood Stem Cell Transplants

In a stem cell transplant, chemotherapy or special medications called growth factors are given to the donor. ■ Sometimes, your child may donate his own stem cells. ■ This treatment forces stem cells to leave the marrow and circulate in the bloodstream. ■ The cells are collected (this is called leukopheresis). ■ Each stem cell collection takes two to three hours, and often the donor is asleep.

The stem cells may be purged of cancer cells and then frozen. ■ Then, like bone marrow transplants, your child receives chemotherapy and/or radiation, and the stem cells are injected back into him. ■ Again, your child stays in hospital until the blood counts have recovered, and he is eating well.

There is increasing interest in obtaining stem cells from the umbilical cords of healthy newborns. ■ Why? ■ The blood from umbilical cords

• contains many stem cells, so we don't need a lot of blood to get a good quantity of them.
• is less likely to cause graft-versus-host disease because a newborn baby hasn't developed a lot of immunity.

While using blood from umbilical cords isn't common practice now, it may be more widely used in the future.

CHAPTER 11 IN BRIEF

Blood cells are produced in the bone marrow, where they grow from "stem" cells and mature by the millions every day. Some blood disorders and cancers are treated by transplanting new bone marrow into children. This bone marrow may be taken from the child himself (perhaps after it has been treated to remove malignant cells) or from a genetically compatible person, sometimes a brother or sister.

If your child is having a bone marrow transplant, he will be treated first with intensive chemotherapy and sometimes radiation. Then, the bone marrow from the donor is injected into him. The donor cells move through the bloodstream and settle in your child's own bone marrow to produce new blood cells.

Stem cells are also found in the bloodstream and may be collected from a donor (by a process much like donating blood). Sometimes, stem cells are obtained from the umbilical cords of healthy newborn babies.

Stem cells are given to your child in the same way as a bone marrow transplant. This is called a blood stem cell transplant. Bone marrow and blood stem cell transplants are simple to do but carry some significant risks to your child's life, including greater susceptibility to serious infection. Despite the risks, transplants are a promising form of treatment for some childhood cancers.

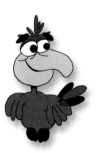

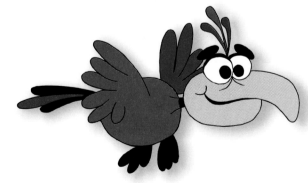

NOTES

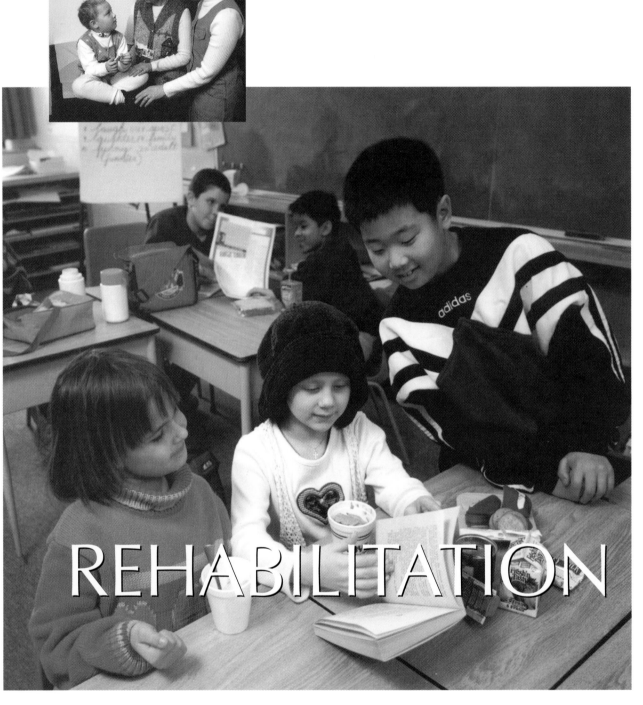

REHABILITATION

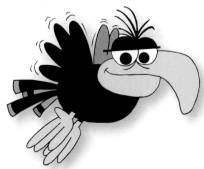

REHABILITATION MEANS HELPING A DISABLED PERSON
CONTINUE A NORMAL LIFE. DISABILITY MEANS LOSING, OR
REDUCING, THE ABILITY TO DO NORMAL DAY-TO-DAY
FUNCTIONS, SUCH AS GETTING AROUND, TAKING CARE OF
ONESELF, GOING TO WORK OR TO SCHOOL, TAKING PART IN
HOBBIES OR OTHER LEISURE ACTIVITIES, AND
MAINTAINING A ROLE IN THE FAMILY.

A child with cancer may have difficulty doing some of these daily functions, either because of the cancer itself or its medical or surgical treatment. ■ For example, leukemia and lymphoma may cause bone and joint pain, which interferes with walking or other activities. ■ Certain tumors can affect nerves, which weakens the muscles. ■ Removing a tumor through surgery may mean losing muscle or bone or both from a limb. ■ Chemotherapy can cause temporary weakness and reduced energy. ■ Radiation therapy may interfere with growth of bone and soft tissues, resulting in unequal limb lengths or curvatures of the spine. ■ It's important to deal with all disabilities with an organized, rehabilitation approach.

The Management Team

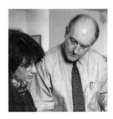

Rehabilitation of any child with a long-term illness includes four components: physical, psychological, social, and educational. ■ A team of people, working closely together, will be involved in looking at all these components. ■ The team may include a pediatric oncologist, surgeon, radiation oncologist, nurse, physiotherapist, social worker, occupational therapist, school teacher, child life specialist, prosthetist, orthotist, speech language pathologist, and nutritionist. ■ You and your child will be at the center of this group's attention.

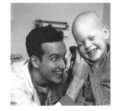

Ideally, the team begins working as soon as your child is diagnosed. ■ The rehabilitation physician will look at how well your child can carry out his daily activities and will develop and supervise a plan for improvement.

All of the health care team members will meet often to talk over your child's rehabilitation, and, if necessary, change the goals and treatment plan. ■ They will also answer any questions or concerns that you or your child may have.

Goals of Rehabilitation

The goals of a rehabilitation program for the child with cancer include

- preventing or limiting any factors that could make the disability more severe or long lasting
- returning your child to his former lifestyle by treating any disability or changing his activity or environment to allow former function to continue

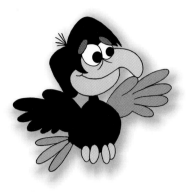

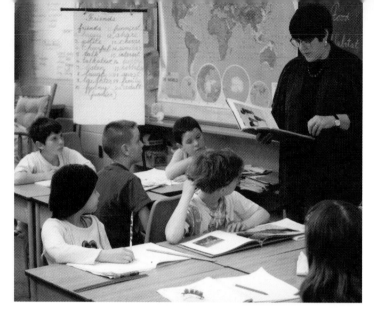

- providing support and education to help you and your child with any stress if the disability is permanent
- preventing complications that may further reduce quality of life or providing equipment or comfort to improve life quality if the cancer can't be cured.

Managing Disabilities

Daily Living: Activities like eating, dressing, cleansing, going to the toilet, and exercising may be more difficult to do or may take much more energy because of pain or tiredness. ■ The occupational therapist can teach your child new ways of doing these activities that will make them easier.

Play: Being able to play is important to your child. ■ Changes to your child's play activities can help him take part more easily, and play can add to, or replace, more structured (and often boring!) exercise routines.

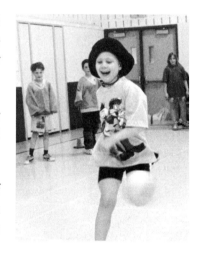

Mobility: Some children lose a leg through surgery. ■ Other forms of treatment, as well as cancer itself, can make it difficult for your child to walk because of bone or joint pain, stiff or contracted joints, loss of muscle strength or even paralysis, loss of sensation, and poor balance.

The physiotherapist can improve your child's ability to move around. Depending on your child's needs, the physiotherapist will teach you and your family some exercises to improve mobility. ■ Your child may need to be taught to walk with

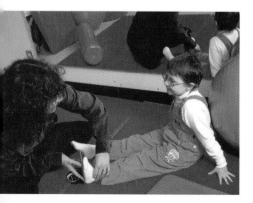

crutches, artificial limbs, braces, or splints. ■ Sometimes, a wheelchair may have to be used temporarily.

Breathing: Cancer or its treatment can sometimes interfere with breathing. ■ If your child's muscles are weak, coughing may be less effective. ■ The immune system may be weak, so your child has a greater chance of getting chest infections. ■ Stiffness in the lung tissues or bone changes can reduce the amount of air that he can move in and out of his lungs. ■ He can be taught breathing and coughing exercises by the physiotherapist to help maintain proper breathing. ■ General

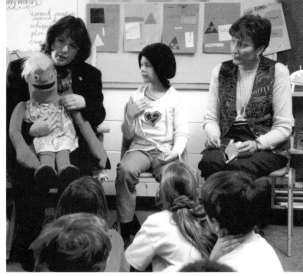

exercise programs help your child use oxygen more efficiently, and back exercises or bracing can help maintain chest volume. ■ If he can't clear secretions from his lungs, there are special techniques that can help, such as postural drainage (which takes advantage of gravity, in different positions, to drain secretions).

Pain: Pain often causes disability in a child with cancer. ■ There are several ways the rehabilitation team can help relieve pain, such as splints, heat, massage, and transcutaneous nerve stimulation. ■ Nerves that supply areas where pain is felt can be blocked by an injection of chemicals or surgically cut. ■ There are also many medications that can help relieve pain.

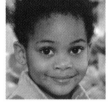

Educating Teachers and Classmates: Although not always possible, every effort should be made to keep your child in his regular classroom. ■ If he has a disability that interferes with activities in the classroom, the occupational therapist can visit the school to assess his needs and make recommendations about special equipment or changes to his program. ■ Sometimes, cancer and its treatment will affect a child's ability to learn. ■ Tests should be done by a psychologist with the school so that the right educational programs can be found. ■ It's important to tell the teacher and classmates about your child's cancer, any disability, and the help he needs. ■ This information can be provided (with your permission) by the clinic nurse, child life specialist, and social worker.

CHAPTER 12 IN BRIEF

As a result of cancer or its treatment, your child may not be able to take part in many of his usual activities. Pain, weakness, fatigue, and difficulty in walking or breathing may interfere with your child's normal functioning. The health care team will be keeping a close eye on his status. Whenever necessary, they will help your child with any physical and emotional challenges and support you in your efforts to return him to a fulfilling lifestyle. By working together, we can improve your child's quality of life throughout his treatment and beyond.

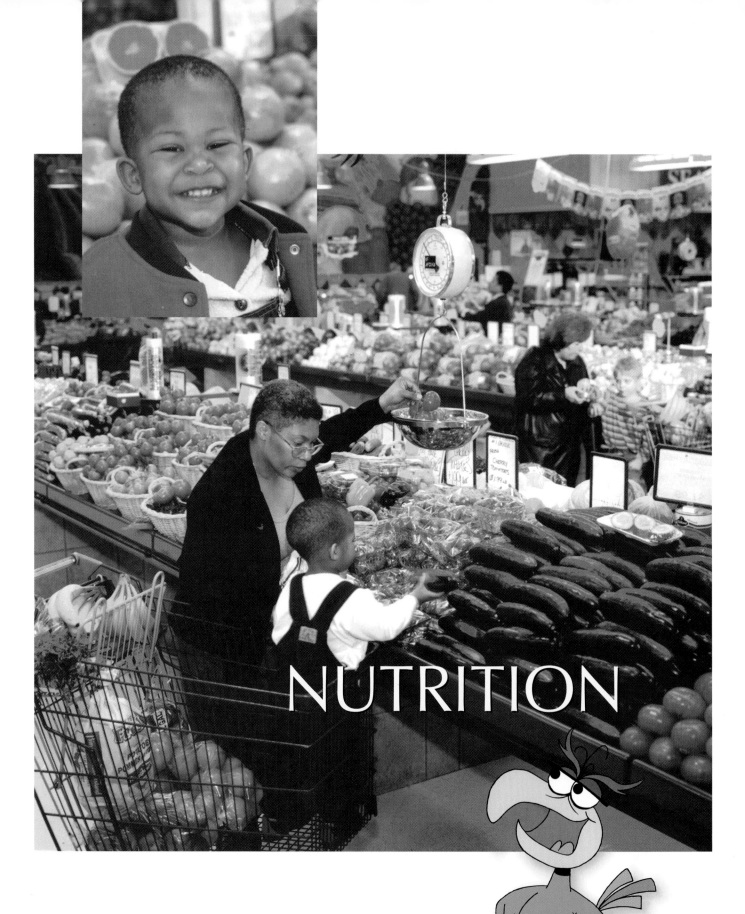

NUTRITION

GOOD NUTRITION IS IMPORTANT FOR ALL CHILDREN, BUT ESPECIALLY FOR THOSE WITH CANCER.

Surgery, chemotherapy, and radiation treatments all increase your child's need for foods that help his body heal and grow. ■ Every child who has chemotherapy, and many who receive radiation, will have some changes in eating habits. ■ Good nutrition can help your child

- not to lose too much weight by keeping reserves of muscle and fat.
- keep to a healthy weight so he can receive the right dosages of drugs.
- have fewer side effects from treatment, such as weakness, lowered immunity, and greater risk of infections.
- recover more quickly from side effects of treatment.
- feel better and have more energy to do "kids' stuff."

Much of the information you will find in books and magazines is about cancer in adults, but this information is not always correct for children. ■ Below is nutritional information relevant to children.

Do certain foods cause cancer?

In adults, we believe there is a link between diet and cancer in some of the most common cancers such as colon and breast cancer. ■ No such link has been found for most cancers in children. ■ **Poor diet is not the cause of childhood cancer.**

Do certain foods prevent cancer?

There is a lot of information suggesting that changing what we eat, such as eating more fruit, vegetables, and high-fiber grains, will protect us from developing cancer. ■ But always remember that prevention is not treatment. ■ Until there is better understanding of how dietary supplements or nutrients (such as antioxidants) affect cancer, they are not recommended in the treatment of children with cancer.

Do certain foods treat cancer?

Anti-cancer foods as such do not exist, but good nutrition is an important part of cancer therapy.

Nutrition Is a Part of Cancer Treatment

Maintaining your child's best nutritional health is an important part of his treatment.

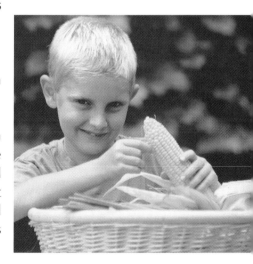

Overall, nutrition is most easily measured by changes in weight and height. ■ Your child's weight and height will be compared to the growth of other children his age. ■ The blood tests your child will have regularly also provide many clues about how food energy is used and whether certain vitamins and minerals are in good supply. ■ These clues will help your child's team to decide about nutritional treatment.

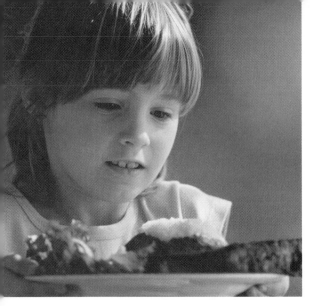

Side effects of cancer treatment include nausea, vomiting, diarrhea, mouth sores, and changes in appetite and taste. ■ As well, many children receiving cancer treatment lose weight because emotional and physical changes affect how they eat.

Nutritional side effects of treatment can be immediate (within hours), intermediate (within days), or long term (lasting even after treatment has finished).

Immediate Side Effects

Immediate side effects of nausea and vomiting are controlled mostly with medications. ■ There are some dietary changes that may help. ■ During these days, your child may complain that foods taste bitter or just taste "funny."

Intermediate Side Effects

Intermediate side effects are the hardest to deal with. ■ This is when you can see the direct effect of the chemotherapy on your child's healthy cells. ■ Blood cell counts fall, and the risk of infection is great. ■ Sore mouth, constipation, or diarrhea may be a problem. ■ Anorexia (an extreme loss of appetite) is common. ■ You might try to give your child his favorite foods and special treats, but he probably won't want them. ■ It's even more frustrating because your child is probably feeling fine otherwise.

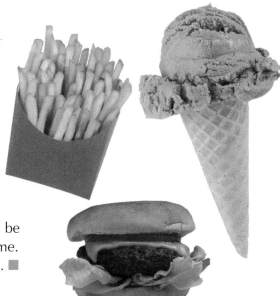

Long-Term Side Effects

Long-term side effects are less common. ■ Overall growth may be affected because a child may have poor nutrition for a long time. ■ Normal eating behaviors are forgotten and difficult to start again. ■ Rarely, there are permanent changes in taste and smell.

The key is to have a relaxed attitude toward eating.

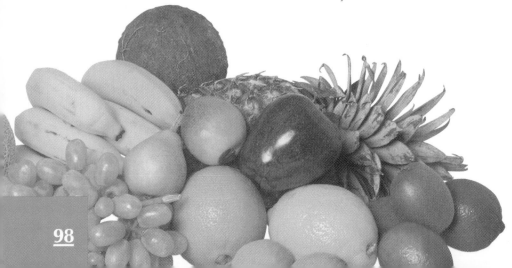

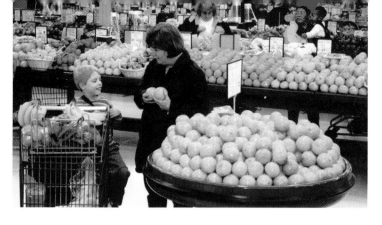
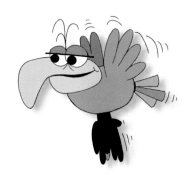

Helping Your Child to Healthy Eating

You can do a lot to help your child eat. ■ Concentrate on improving how much and how well he eats. ■ This approach works best during times when your child is eating well.

Food Safety

Sometimes, food can be unsafe to eat because bacteria grow in it. ■ You may not be able to see, taste, or smell these bacteria, but they can be harmful to people who have a weak immune system. ■ Bacteria grow quickly between 4°C to 60°C/40°F to 140°F. ■ To keep foods safe, shorten the length of time the food is sitting within this temperature range.

When grocery shopping,

- buy cans or jars without dents, cracks, bulges, and leaks.
- make sure eggs aren't cracked or broken.
- shop for your meats last and put them in plastic bags. This prevents the juices from getting on your hands or anything else in your cart.
- check "best before" dates on dairy products and don't buy items at or near this date.
- buy foods such as meat and cheese that are packaged on the day that you buy them.
- pick up your hot and cold foods toward the end of your shopping.
- after you finish shopping, return home and refrigerate cold food quickly. Cold and hot foods should never be kept at room temperature longer than two hours.

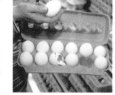

Keeping your kitchen clean can help lower the amount of bacteria.

When preparing food,

- wash your hands with soap and water before touching it.
- use plastic cutting boards instead of wooden boards. Bacteria can grow in the wooden grooves.
- wash all utensils, boards, countertops, and appliances with hot, soapy water before and after contact with raw food items.
- wash fruits and vegetables well with water.

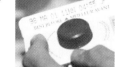

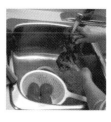

When you're cooking,

- thaw foods in the refrigerator or in the microwave, never on the kitchen counter.
- if microwaving, follow temperature and cooking time recommendations.
- if barbecuing, pre-cook meats to make sure meats are well done.
- do not use slow cookers. In slow cookers, food is cooked for a long time at temperatures ideal for bacteria to grow.
- cook meats, poultry, fish, and eggs so they are well done.

When you store food,

- divide large amounts of leftovers into small, shallow containers for quick cooling in the refrigerator.
- keep raw foods, such as meat, chicken, and fish, away from ready-to-eat foods. You can do this by putting these foods in their own containers or plastic bags.
- Throw out moldy food.
- Store leftovers in the refrigerator no longer than 24 hours.

When eating out,

- order meats, poultry, fish, and eggs well done.
- do not order items that have raw food in them, such as caesar salad, sushi, mousses, and hollandaise sauce.
- make sure the salad bar or seafood bar is clean, and all food is on ice.
- do not buy from street vendors.
  - if you are not sure how the food is cooked, ask.

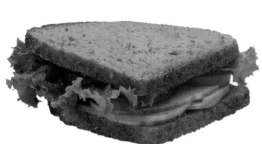

Healthy Eating: What You and Your Child Can Do

- Knowing how children eat can make your job easier.
- Most children don't eat like their parents. Instead, your child likely eats throughout the day and has many small snacks.
- What your child eats is more important than how much he eats.
- How much your child eats is more important than when it is eaten.
- Making mealtimes enjoyable is as important as making sure the food is nutritious.

The most common problems that parents face at home are nausea, decreased appetite, and changes in taste. ■ In hospital, the nutritionist and your child's nurse will keep a watch on how well your child is eating. ■ When your child is an outpatient, you need to keep your child's health care team informed about his eating. ■ Problems will be less upsetting if you can set some goals and develop a plan when your child isn't eating. ■ The nutritionist will be able to meet with you to help as your child's nutritional needs change.

It is your job to offer nutritious foods to your child in an enjoyable atmosphere. It is your child's job to eat as best he can.

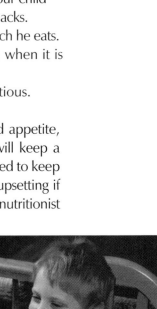

Help your child to know that you will not cater to his every food whim. ■ Fights about food and eating, overwhelming sadness, and busy mealtimes are some of the things that get in the way of your child eating. ■ When eating is difficult, it is important for your child to hear that he is doing okay.

Good Eating Tips

- Recognize your child's efforts, no matter how small. Rewards for good eating behavior will help your child to keep working at eating.

- Don't refuse dessert in an effort to make your child eat good foods. Try small desserts for small meals or offer healthy desserts.
- Food "jags"—picking the same foods repeatedly for days—are common in childhood. Let your child eat these foods instead of fighting about it.
- Allow your child to dislike some foods.
- Make each mouthful count. Most foods can be made more healthy by adding extra energy (calories) as sugar or fat. This way, you can make one meal for your family to enjoy together.
  - Make room for healthy snacks such as milk, juice, yogurt, cheese, fruit, ice cream, or cookies. These foods contain calories and nutrients such as protein, vitamins, and minerals. Try having a special cupboard or basket in the fridge, where your child knows to find food when he is hungry.
    - Only offer your child three or four choices. You and your child may hope that by hitting upon the right food, he will be able to eat more, but too many choices can be confusing.

Mild weight loss

To help your child lose as little weight as possible, make each mouthful count!

- Offer him smaller portion sizes more often. Have a specific schedule so your child will know when meals will happen. This will stimulate his appetite and reduce the stress of being nagged about eating.
- Don't use low-calorie substitutes when you are cooking or preparing food.
- Offer smaller portions of filling foods at mealtime. Low-fat, starchy foods, like potatoes, pasta, rice, and breads, are good choices.

Encourage high-fat foods (with the advice of a nutritionist or dietitian).

- Fry foods instead of using low-fat cooking methods like baking, boiling, broiling, steaming, or microwaving.
- Use higher-fat cold cuts such as bologna and salami.
- Try nuts and peanut butter more often.
- Use butter, oil, margarine, mayonnaise, sour cream, and salad dressings as much as you can. Avoid light varieties with less fat.
  - Snack foods, such as potato chips and corn chips, are high in fat, salt, and calories. Cookies, cakes, pastries, chocolate bars, and candy add extra sugar, fat, and calories. When these foods are the only ones your child will eat, they are important in keeping him nourished.

Nausea and vomiting

This is a time to avoid favorite foods. 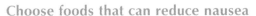 Bad associations can happen easily between favorite foods and the sick feeling your child has on chemotherapy days.

- Save the foods your child enjoys the most for times when he is eating well.
- Ask friends and family to bring food treats for your child to you at home or when your child is not having chemotherapy.
- Strong food smells can be upsetting. ■ When possible, keep your child away from cooking odors.
- At home, he may prefer to stay away from the kitchen when meals are being prepared.
- In hospital, remove the cover from your child's tray before it enters the room. Try offering your child drinks in a lidded cup.
- Cold foods have less upsetting aromas. Popsicles, gelatin desserts, custards, dry cereals, toast, or yogurt may go down better.

Plan ahead

- Try to get your child to eat small amounts frequently.
- Offer your child food every two to three hours, even if he eats only a mouthful.
- Between times, occupy your child with other things and avoid talking about food or having your child watch others eating.
- After eating, encourage your child not to lie down for at least 30 minutes. Plan a game or activity that he can do in an upright position to give time to help with digestion.

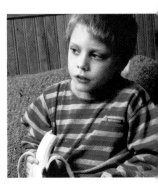

Choose foods that can reduce nausea

- High-fat foods, such as fried or snack foods, take longer to digest and may worsen nausea.
- Fluid is especially important if your child is vomiting. If your child at home is not able to drink six to 10 cups of fluid per day and keep it down, you should contact the clinic.

Mouth problems

- Try to get your child to regularly use mouthwashes and take care of his teeth and gums.

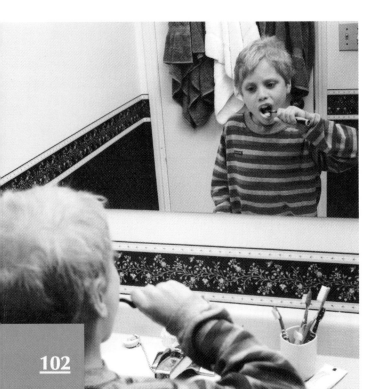

- Avoid hot foods. Your child may find cold or room temperature foods less irritating.
- Avoid salty, spicy, or rough foods.
- Try some soft-textured foods before problems develop. Together with your child, make a list of easy-to-swallow foods to try at times when swallowing hurts. Experiment with foods put in the blender. Try pureed or baby food added to soup or milkshakes. Dunk or soak dry foods in liquids. Use extra butter (or margarine), gravies, sauces, dressings, yogurt, or applesauce to moisten foods.
- Offer your child drinks through a straw. He may find swallowing easier if he tips his head backwards or forwards with each mouthful.

Constipation

- Fluid, especially with high-fiber foods, is the best way to prevent constipation. Juices, such as prune juice and apple juice, will help even more.
- Encourage your child to eat more high-fiber foods. Choose foods made from grains or add regular bran, bran flakes, or bran buds to your cooking. Bran can be added to any foods you would otherwise prepare with oatmeal, breadcrumbs, or flour, such as pancakes, baked goods, meatloaf, and hamburgers.
- Medications for constipation are often needed during chemotherapy. Your child's pharmacist or doctor will tell you how often and how long to use them.
- Make special plans to do daily exercise with your child, such as walking, running, or standing. It will help constipation and keep your child's bones healthy during chemotherapy.

Weight gain

Weight gain, in most cases, is a good thing. ■ It usually means that treatment is becoming less severe and that your child is feeling well. ■ However, too much weight gain is not good.

The most common cause of too much weight gain is a drug called prednisone. ■ This drug affects how your child controls his appetite and how his body uses food energy. ■ Weight gain is caused by retained water and increase in body fat. ■ This weight gain happens quickly and usually doesn't last. ■ The best way to keep your child's weight to a good level is to give lower-energy (calorie) substitutes.

- Don't cut out. Cut back. Offer your child smaller portion sizes, cutting back little by little.
- Try low-calorie substitutes when you are cooking or preparing food. Use yogurt instead of sour cream in dips. Use skim or 1 percent milk instead of whole milk.
- Offer more filling foods at mealtime. Low-fat, starchy foods, like potatoes, pasta, rice, and breads, are good choices.

Watch out for hidden fat in foods.
- Use low-fat cooking methods. Baking, boiling, broiling, steaming, or microwaving is better than frying.
- Use low-fat cold cuts such as lean ham, roast beef, chicken, and turkey.
- Offer nuts and peanut butter less often.
- Use small amounts of butter, oil, margarine, mayonnaise, sour cream, and salad dressings. Try light varieties with less fat.
- Avoid snack foods such as potato chips and corn chips. These foods are high in fat, salt, and calories.
- Avoid cookies, cakes, pastries, chocolate bars, and candy. These foods add extra sugar, fat, and calories to your child's diet.

When Nutritional Support Is Needed

It's okay for your child's weight to vary in small amounts, but when he loses more than 10 percent of his weight over 6 months, specialized nutritional support, in the form of tube feeding or total parenteral nutrition (TPN), is needed to prevent more weight loss.

Specialized nutritional support is used only after all efforts to improve your child's voluntary eating have been tried. ■ Your input is important in making the decision to put your child on nutritional support.

Tube Feeding

When your child won't eat because he doesn't have an appetite, voluntary eating can be "beefed up" by dripping nutrients directly into his stomach. ■ This may be done using a small, soft tube that is passed into the stomach through your child's nose. ■ Tube feeding is important when we know that side effects of treatment will be severe.

Tube feeding can be started in the clinic or as an inpatient. ■ Usually, your child will be admitted to hospital for a few days to get started and give you time to learn how to manage the feedings at home. ■ Placing the tube takes about five minutes. ■ The child life specialist can help your child deal with any stress and fear about having the tube put in and will teach him some tips to make insertion easier. ■ Your child can eat or drink as usual with the tube in place. ■ At first, he will feel the tube in place and may find it unpleasant, but in about a day, he will get used to it.

Ready-made formula is used for tube feeding. ■ The formula is put into your child slowly using a pump, much like those used for intravenous solutions. ■ In hospital, you will learn how to operate the pump, set up and clean the equipment, and remove the feeding tube in an emergency. ■ Some children and their families decide to remove and replace the tube every day so that feeding is done overnight and the child is free of the tube during the day. ■ For most children, it is safe to keep the same tube in place for one month. ■ This choice is up to you. ■ When you feel comfortable using this equipment, you are ready to go home. ■ You may be able to get financial assistance for home nutritional therapy. ■ There are a number of programs available. ■ Ask your home care co-ordinator, nutritionist, or social worker.

A tube called a gastrostomy is used if tube feeding will last more than a month or so. ■ This tube is placed from the outside of the belly into the stomach during an operation. ■ This allows tube feeding directly into the gut so that a tube into the nose isn't needed. ■ New types of gastrostomy tubes, which can be put in about a month after the first one, have no external tube, so your child can wear snug-fitting clothes or swim.

Tube feeding and gastrostomy feeding can greatly improve your child's quality of living. ■ He can enjoy mealtime with the family without the guilt of not being able to eat well.

Total parenteral nutrition

At times when your child can neither eat nor take tube feeding, intravenous nutrition is used. ■ With TPN, the gut is not used. ■ Instead, all of the nutrients enter the body through a vein. ■ Most often, this is done using your child's right atrial catheter (see Chapter 7). ■ Unlike tube feeding, TPN cannot be done easily at home.

Special Diets for Some Chemotherapy

Prednisone or other steroids: low-sodium diet

When your child is receiving prednisone or other steroid drugs, he may need to be on a low-sodium diet. ■ Sodium is a mineral found in all living cells. ■ It is present naturally in your body and in the foods you eat. ■ Normally, the level of sodium found in your body is controlled by the kidneys. ■ Prednisone, like other steroids, changes this control, and your body keeps too much sodium, which causes the body to hold fluid. ■ Sometimes, this leads to high blood pressure. ■ Reducing sodium in the diet helps the body to get rid of fluid.

The major source of sodium in your diet is table salt (sodium chloride). ■ Baking soda, baking powder, preserved and convenience foods, and medications such as antacids, effervescent salts, and some laxatives can also contain large amounts of sodium.

Don't add salt at the table, although small amounts may be used in cooking. ■ Salt substitutes and sea salt should not be used.

Your child may choose only one of the following high-salt foods per day:

Breads and cereals
Salted crackers such as Triscuits, Ritz Crackers, soda crackers with salted tops, pretzels, and other salted snack foods, commercially prepared breading products (e.g., Shake 'n' Bake), and waffle and pancake mixes.

Meat and alternatives
Smoked, salted, cured, and pickled meats, or poultry or fish such as bacon, corned beef, wieners, sausage, ham, luncheon meats, processed cheese slices, and cheese spreads, purchased breaded or battered meats, or fish products, canned meats, and convenience foods.

Other foods
Ketchup, chili sauce, soy sauce, prepared mustard, Worcestershire sauce, gravy base, pickles and relish, seasoned salts and MSG, certain mineral waters, snack foods such as potato chips, salted popcorn, and salted nuts.

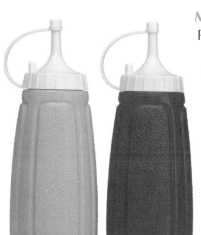

Mixed foods and casseroles
Pizza, commercial macaroni and cheese.

Fruit and vegetables
Artificial fruit-flavored crystals, brine-cured vegetables such as sauerkraut, pickled vegetables, canned vegetables such as canned tomatoes, stewed tomatoes, and tomato sauce.

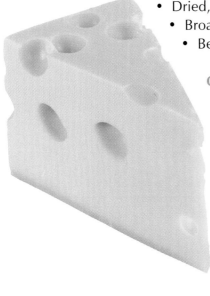

Soup

Bouillon, meat extracts, dry soup mixes or instant soup (e.g., Cup-a-Soup), beef or chicken cubes, and regular canned soup.

Fats

Bacon fat, commercial salad dressings, salad and vegetable dips made with dehydrated mixes.

Desserts

Commercial cakes and pastries.

Procarbazine: MAOI diet

Procarbazine is a drug used to treat cancer such as Hodgkin's disease. ■ One of the side effects of this drug can be high blood pressure and headaches. ■ Procarbazine stops the breakdown of certain brain chemicals, including the chemical tyramine, found in many foods.

To avoid this serious complication, it is important that your child avoid foods that are high in tyramine. ■ A low-tyramine diet is also called the MAOI or monoamine oxidase inhibitor diet. ■ Your child will need to follow this diet while he is taking procarbazine and for two weeks after stopping the drug. ■ Plan meals carefully to offer the following restricted foods in between procarbazine treatments.

Avoid these foods:

- Aged cheese—cheese and cheese dishes such as pizza, lasagna, and macaroni and cheese. Cream cheese, cottage cheese, and ricotta cheese are allowed.
- Dry sausage such as salami, pepperoni, summer sausage, and mortadella
- Sauerkraut
- Yeast extracts such as brewer's yeast or Marmite
- Dried, smoked, or pickled fish
- Broad bean pods such as fava beans, lima beans
- Beer and wine

Other hints:

- Do not use cold remedies or cough medications.
- Use only small amounts of overripe fruits such as bananas, banana breads, or muffins.
- Each day, your child may have a maximum of two 250-mL (8-ounce) serving drinks containing caffeine such as cola, tea, or coffee.
- Food freshness is important. Don't offer your child food if you're not sure about its freshness. Only fresh, freshly canned, or frozen food should be used. Check expiry dates on foods carefully.
- Thaw foods only in the refrigerator. Do not thaw foods at room temperature. Do not use leftovers after one to two days.

Methotrexate and dietary folate

Methotrexate is a drug that interferes with the way the body uses a vitamin called folate. ■ For this reason, it is important that your child not have too much folate in his diet when this drug is given.

- Always have your child's doctor, pharmacist, or nutritionist have a look at any vitamin/mineral preparation before giving it to your child.
- Preparations available through health food stores and alternative health care practitioners often contain unknown amounts of a number of substances. Tissue extracts, "high-potency" tablets, and "immuneboosters" may contain large amounts of folate. Any one of these may interfere with your child's treatment. Ask your child's health care team to have a look at all of these preparations before your child takes them.

Complementary and Alternative Therapies

It is natural to find out all you can do about your child's health and cancer treatment. When your child is bothered by side effects, you may want to experiment with other kinds of treatments. ■ Often, this means thinking about alternative approaches. ■ Some families consult "alternative" health practitioners such as naturopaths, homeopaths, and herbalists. ■ Complementary therapies, although untested, are used by parents along with conventional therapies. ■ Alternative therapies are used instead of conventional treatment.

This section will not discuss the details about specific complementary or alternative therapies. ■ Members of your health care team can talk to you about different cancer treatment approaches. ■ Review with them some of your own research in this area. ■ **It is vital that you discuss any changes in your child's diet with the team.** ■ This section is designed to help you make good decisions about other kinds of treatments.

How do I know if the treatment is safe for my child?

When considering whether to start complementary cancer treatment for your child, consider the following:

- Has the therapy been proven to be more effective than doing nothing?
- Is it as safe as doing nothing?
- Is the potential benefit greater than the potential harm to your child or to your family?
- Have the people who support this treatment proven that the treatment is safe and effective in an acceptable manner?

If you can't answer yes to all of these questions, your child's health care team may not support your decision to go ahead with treatment. ■ However, your child will still receive the conventional treatment.

Complementary therapy is okay if

- it doesn't do any harm; in other words, it doesn't interfere with drugs being used to treat your child, and it doesn't cost your family too much money.
- it's not used as a substitute for proven, conventional cancer treatment.
- it provides the right nutrition for your growing child.

However, there are some concerns about many of the complementary treatments now available. ■ Some of these treatments may be unsafe, and none of them has been shown in a scientific way to do what they claim to do. ■ With the best intentions, some parents give supplements to their child that are actually harmful to them. ■ "Nutritional advice" from those who are not directly involved in cancer care should always be checked with the people who specialize in treating cancer. ■ Naturopaths may be able to advise on a variety of health issues, but they don't have proper training in cancer and may give the wrong information to cancer patients and their families.

Why are alternative treatments different from standard treatments?

The term "alternative" implies that an unproven treatment is as good as or better than standard, medical treatments. ■ There is not enough evidence to make such a statement, and there are a growing number of alternative treatments for cancer that haven't been proven by scientific studies.

Unproven therapies commonly

- offer a cure.
- are promoted for general use. In other words, they are for all patients, regardless of their age, type of disease, stage of disease, or success with other treatments. They are not individualized to your needs. Unlike the treatment that your child is receiving, no studies have been done to see if the alternative approach is effective in treating your child's cancer.
- have been prescribed without knowing your child's medical history, disease, and reaction to treatment and without knowing about the experience from many children with the same illness.

The standard treatment your child receives is the most effective we know about right now. You can be confident of this because

- animal and laboratory tests have shown that the treatment is effective and as safe as it can be.
- there is evidence it has helped children with the same cancer that your child has.
- testing has been done on large enough numbers of children to be certain that the effects aren't just a matter of chance.

The use of alternative as distinct from complementary approaches is not supported by your health care team when active conventional therapy has been planned or initiated.

CHAPTER 13 IN BRIEF

Good nutrition is essential for children undergoing or recovering from cancer treatment. If your child is well nourished, he will tolerate therapy better and recover faster. But the side effects of treatment—like nausea, vomiting, diarrhea, constipation, mouth sores, and changes in appetite—can get in the way of good nutrition.

It's normal to be concerned about weight loss and lack of appetite in your child, but remember that these things are not unusual in children having cancer treatment. Try not to become obsessive or confrontational with your child about eating. Instead, have realistic expectations and be flexible in planning meals; for instance, offer high-fat, high-calorie foods to encourage weight gain and appetite. Be sure to take full advantage of the nutritionist's knowledge and experience.

Be cautious about "complementary" or "alternative" treatments for cancer. They can be costly, ineffective, and, more importantly, may interfere with treatments of proven value given at the hospital. Always talk to your child's doctor first before trying any "alternative" options.

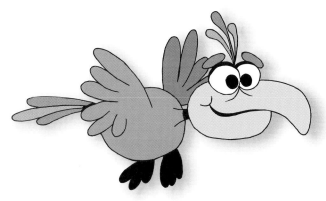

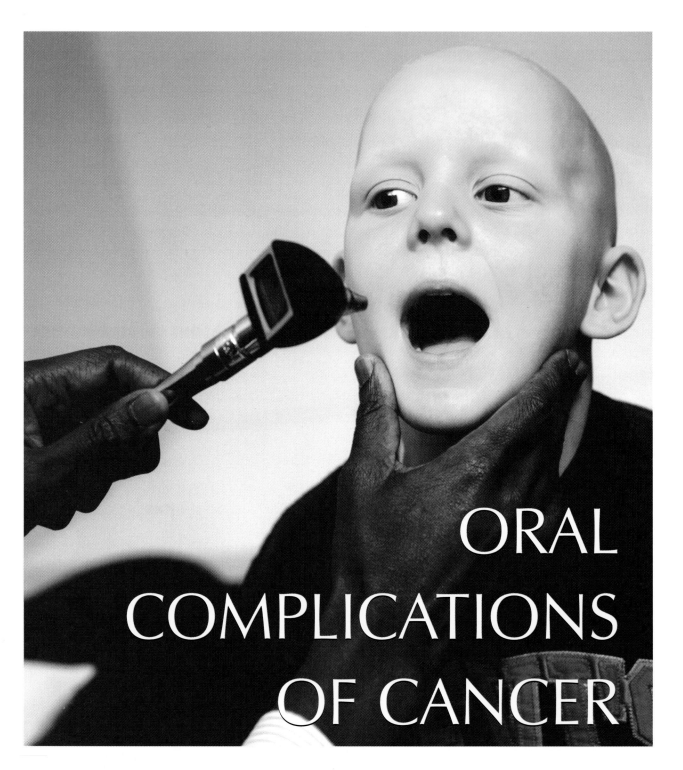

ORAL
COMPLICATIONS
OF CANCER
IN CHILDREN

PROBLEMS CAN DEVELOP IN YOUR CHILD'S MOUTH EITHER DUE TO THE CANCER OR ITS TREATMENT.

These problems include mucositis, when the lining of the mouth (mucosa) becomes red and tender, sores (ulceration), and infections and bleeding in the mouth.

Effects of Chemotherapy

Cells grow rapidly in places like the lining of the mouth, making this area sensitive to cancer drugs. ■ The lining of the mouth can become thinner, resulting in mucositis and ulceration. ■ This usually happens on the floor of the mouth, but the cheeks and the side of and underneath the tongue can be affected too.

Chemotherapy can also cause a decrease in saliva, which might make it difficult for your child to swallow, eat, and speak. ■ Without enough saliva, the bacteria in the mouth grow more rapidly, and cavities may develop in teeth.

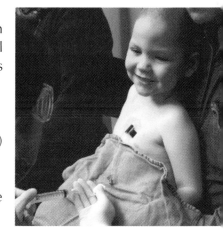

As we discussed in Chapter 7, chemotherapy can interfere with the production of bone marrow, which can lead to abnormal bleeding and a lowered resistance to infection. ■ Signs of this bleeding can be seen in the mouth

- as round, red patches on the inside of the cheeks
- at gum margins (where the teeth meet the gums)
- in places where trauma has occurred (for example, tongue-biting)
- with recent tooth removals.

Sometimes, severe infections can result from dental problems like gum disease and decayed or damaged teeth.

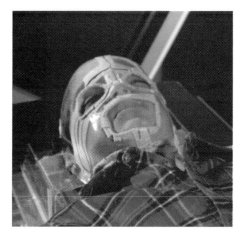

Effects of Radiotherapy

Radiation can damage the lining of the mouth, salivary glands, muscles of chewing, developing teeth, and surrounding bone. ■ Signs of this damage include mucositis, dry mouth, muscle spasms, many cavities, infections in the mouth, and dental and facial growth abnormalities.

How to Prevent or Lessen Problems in the Mouth

A dental examination is done as early as possible to identify and treat any dental problems that might cause difficulties once treatment begins. ■ Teeth that are badly decayed or infected will be removed. ■ This is particularly important if your child is having radiotherapy to his head and neck or is having a bone marrow transplant. ■ It's also important that any broken teeth, fillings, or sharp areas from braces be removed or corrected as soon as possible so they can't irritate the lining of the mouth.

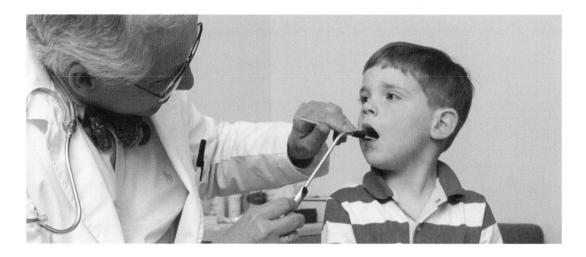

Bacteria from areas of inflammation or sores in the mouth can spread to the rest of the body. ■ To avoid this, you and your child can do several things:

- Try to prevent cuts or other damage to the lips, tongue, and cheeks.
- Brush teeth with ultra-soft bristles and oral sponges three times per day within 20 minutes after meals and before bedtime.
- Use mouth rinses.

If your child has a dry mouth because of a decrease in saliva, there are many mouth rinses that can remove food that causes tooth decay. ■ These include normal saline, 3 percent hydrogen peroxide (diluted), and sodium bicarbonate. ■ Don't use commercial mouth rinses as they can dry the inside of the mouth and increase the chances of getting an injury.

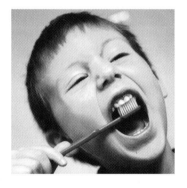

There are also mouthwashes that get rid of bacteria. A 0.2 percent chlorhexidine solution or brush-on gel (used two times per day) reduces bacteria and infections. ■ Sugar-free rinses and swallow mixtures of nystatin also protect against some infections. ■ It's not a good idea to use chlorhexidine and nystatin at the same time as they interfere with each other.

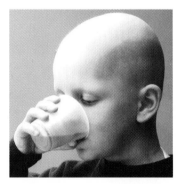

To prevent cavities, your child may also use sodium fluoride rinses (0.05 percent) or brush-on gel (0.4 percent) two to three times per day.

Taking proper care of your child's mouth depends on his age and if he cooperates. ■ You may need to do it for him or, at least, supervise while he is doing it to ensure that it is done properly. ■ If rinsing is not possible, solutions can be swabbed around the mouth with a special sponge or brushed on the teeth with the gel.

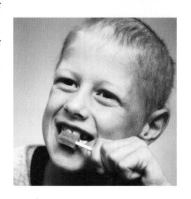

Managing Dry Mouth

To relieve the discomfort of dry mouth,

- offer your child sugar-free gum or candies.
- apply an anesthetic to make eating easier—for example, 2 percent xylocaine gel.
- give your child moist foods and lots of fluids to help in chewing.

Long-Term Dental Problems

Since cancer therapy affects all cells, children may develop problems in their tooth enamel and root structure. ■ The age of a child who develops cancer is important. ■ When children under 10 (whose teeth and gums are developing) are diagnosed with cancer, they may have more long-term dental problems than those children older than 10 years of age. ■ The younger children may have missing teeth, discolored or softer enamel, and thin, stunted roots. ■ These children may need frequent visits to the dentist, braces, and artificial teeth.

CHAPTER 14 IN BRIEF

The mouth is sensitive to the effects of cancer, and painful ulcers may develop as a result. These sores will heal in time but can be uncomfortable in the meantime. Your child may need to be admitted to hospital so the pain can be managed with intravenous medication.

During cancer treatment, good mouth care is vital. That means visiting the dentist regularly, using prescribed mouth rinses and brushing after every meal. If dental work is needed, your child must be given an antibiotic before the procedure to prevent infection. Ask your child's clinic nurse or doctor for more information about smart dental care during cancer treatment.

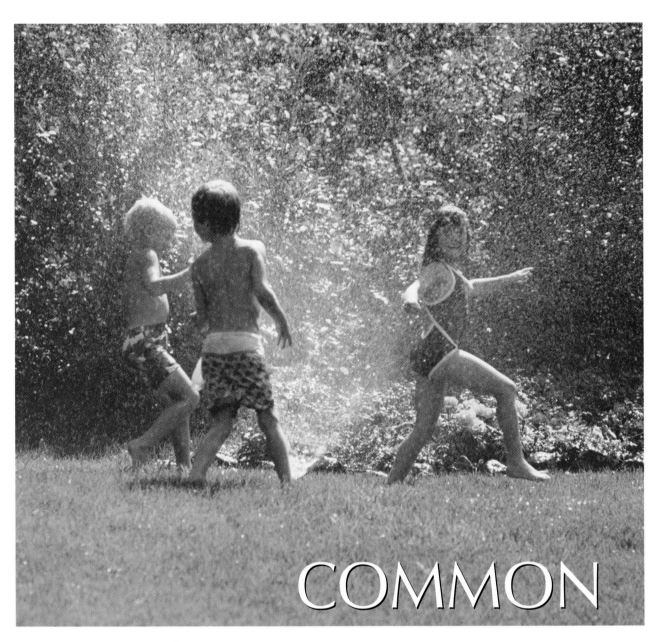

COMMON
CONCERNS

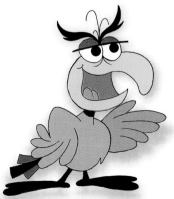

ONE OF OUR MOST IMPORTANT GOALS IS TO HELP YOUR CHILD DEVELOP AND GROW, PHYSICALLY, MENTALLY, AND SOCIALLY.

Growth and Development

There may be special circumstances, such as surgery or radiation therapy, that interrupt normal development. ■ Although development may be slowed down or even go back, most children will eventually catch up. ■ Eventually, most children achieve the same milestones of childhood that all children do. ■ To make sure that your child is progressing as he should, a child life specialist will help keep an eye on him.

School

It's vital that your child attend school and keep up with his school work. ■ If he has missed some school, your clinic nurse will be happy to arrange a school visit to help the teacher and classmates, and your child return. ■ Children with cancer who are attending school have a greater chance of being exposed to illnesses, so staff in school should be aware of the following:

- Your child is vulnerable to chicken pox. ■ The school should tell you if your child has been exposed to someone with chicken pox. ■ If that's the case, tell the clinic immediately. ■ If there is an outbreak of chicken pox in the school, your child should stay home until the peak is over. ■ The school should ask other parents to tell them if they think or know that a child has chicken pox.
- Your child will have side effects from his cancer therapy. ■ For example, if he is taking prednisone, he may have mood swings. ■ It will be important that his teacher understand why he is reacting in unusual ways.
- Your child should be encouraged to take part in regular school activities. ■ If for any reason he should not do a particular activity, the clinic staff will tell you.
- If your child has a right atrial catheter, special precautions may need to be taken. ■ See Chapter 7 for more details.

Emotional Health

Cancer and its treatment will affect your child, not only physically but emotionally too. ■ He may be upset when his normal activities are interrupted or if he has to stay in hospital. ■ You and the rest of your family will be affected too. ■ A positive, healthy mental attitude will not cure cancer, but it may help with your and your child's well-being. ■ See Chapter 3 for more information.

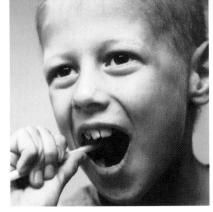

Basic Health Care

As discussed in Chapter 14, proper mouth care is vital. ■ Teeth should be cleaned with a soft toothbrush at least twice a day. ■ Rinsing with a regular or prescribed medicated mouthwash should also be done often each day. ■ This can be done to a young child or infant by wrapping a soft cloth soaked in mouthwash around the finger and wiping his mouth, teeth, and gums. ■ If mouth ulcers or sores develop, cleaning should be done more often. ■ Your child may need a prescribed medication to treat infection. ■ Your child should see a dentist regularly after you have talked to the clinic staff and have dental work when his blood counts permit. ■ If he doesn't have a regular dentist, the clinic staff can refer you to one. ■ The dentist and physician should work together to plan the necessary dental work.

As with all children, a stable, sensible, well-balanced diet is important for growth and development. ■ At times, your child may not want to eat because he has no appetite or has mouth sores. ■ At these times, you and your child will need to work together to ensure he is getting proper nutrition. ■ See Chapter 13 for some useful tips.

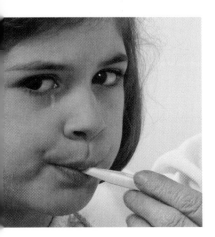

Infections

Normal, healthy children have many upper airway and ear infections every year. ■ The child with cancer has a greater chance of getting bacterial infections when he doesn't have enough white blood cells (neutropenia). ■ You can't prevent all infections, but there are things you can do to prevent many of them:

- Keep your child away from anyone who has an infection.
- When he is neutropenic, avoid crowds, such as in shopping centers.
- Call the clinic immediately if your child develops a fever over 38°C/100°F, other signs of infection, or is exposed to chicken pox, shingles, or hepatitis. ■ For more information on this subject, see Chapter 9, "Infection and the Child with Cancer."

Medications

The drugs prescribed for your child have to be taken according to instructions given by your health care team. ■ It can be hard to remember when and which pills have to be taken, especially when the drug and dose change often, but it is your responsibility to make sure the correct drugs are given at the correct time. ■ If you don't, your child's treatment may not be successful. ■ His doctors, nurses, and pharmacists will help set up the easiest schedule to follow at home. ■ If you forget to give him some of his medications, tell the clinic staff so adjustments can be made to the drug schedule.

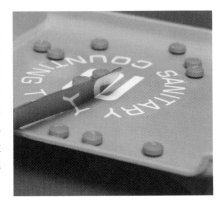

While your child is taking medications at home, it's important that some other drugs be avoided. ■ These include certain products for coughs, colds, and allergies. ■ All products containing acetylsalicylic acid (ASA, aspirin) should be avoided. ■ Tylenol is a better choice as long as your child is not allergic to it. ■ Check with the clinic first before buying any drugs, prescription or non-prescription (including vitamins). ■ Most importantly, remember to always check the label before giving any medications to your child.

Unconventional/Complementary/Alternative Therapy

We are open to suggestions and discussion of other forms of treatment. ■ Many families hear or read about "cures" for cancer. ■ Such forms of "therapy" may or may not be helpful. ■ If you wish to try such approaches, discuss the information with the clinic staff. ■ If an unconventional form of management will not harm your child or interrupt his regular therapy, it may not be discouraged. ■ However, this "treatment" will not be provided by the clinic staff.

Communication

The clinic staff has access to many health professionals, including nutritionists, physiotherapists, dentists, surgeons, and psychologists. ■ The clinic staff can refer you and your child to these people. ■ If your child sees other similar professionals in the community, they must be told about his illness and therapy. ■ For example, if he needs his tonsils removed, the surgeon must be told about the increased risk of bleeding and infection. ■ Your role in sharing information about your child is vital. ■ Of course, your family doctor will also be involved in the care of your child. ■ The clinic will send letters regularly about your child's progress to your family doctor.

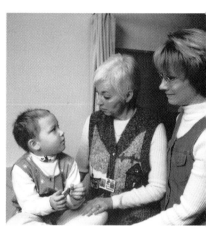

Other Health Care Issues

• Health insurance

If medical coverage for drugs and supplies is not sufficient, tell the clinic staff. ■ They may be able to provide other coverage or give you the information to have coverage extended.

• Life insurance

The prospects for survival of children with cancer continue to improve, so the expectations of these children for life insurance are increasing.

An application for insurance from a survivor of childhood cancer could consist of a signed declaration outlining details of the cancer investigation, diagnosis, and management. ■ The insurer would then request a physician's report on details of tumor stage, cell type, pathology report, types of treatment, response to therapy, and duration of disease-free follow-up.

The final insurance offer to the survivor of childhood cancer would depend on the anticipated death rate for the particular medical condition, the type of policy applied for, and the company's policy about uncommon medical conditions. ■ It's a good idea for the survivor of childhood cancer to shop around to various companies for the best offer.

• ID bracelets

It may be a good idea for your child to wear a medical identification bracelet. ■ If so, you can get information about obtaining a bracelet from the clinic staff.

• Vacations

When planning a vacation, tell the clinic staff well in advance so your child's treatment can be rescheduled and arrangements made for medications and supplies. ■ Always carry with you a letter explaining your child's condition.

When to Contact the Clinic

Always contact the clinic if your child
- has been exposed to or develops chicken pox or another infection.
- is neutropenic (neutrophil count less than 1,000 per cu. mm or 1×10^9/L) and develops a fever or is generally unwell.
- has a normal blood count but develops a fever that doesn't go away or worsens.
- vomits more than usual.
- bleeds—signs of bleeding including bruises, black stools, and pink urine.
- has persistent pain anywhere in his body.
- is due to receive a vaccination (immunization).
- is going to have dental work.
- develops any redness or swelling on any part of his body.
- develops shortness of breath or appears to be having difficulty breathing.
- develops mouth sores and has problems eating or drinking.

How to Contact the Clinic

There is a doctor from the clinic on call 24 hours a day, seven days a week. ■ Call the hospital paging system to contact the right person on statutory holidays, weekends, and after hours. ■ During clinic hours, you can call the receptionist in the clinic.

CHAPTER 15 IN BRIEF

Helping your child feel normal—both physically and mentally—during cancer treatment is essential. Your child should continue to feel an important member of his family and community because, when he recovers from his illness, he will have to deal with life's challenges just like everyone else.

Tell teachers, extended family, and friends about your child's cancer, its treatment, and side effects, and inform them of any special needs he may have. Unless people know, they won't know how to help.

Children with cancer need to go to school, take vacations, and play as they did before their illness. As a parent, do what you can to maintain an active and safe lifestyle for your child during his treatment.

NOTES

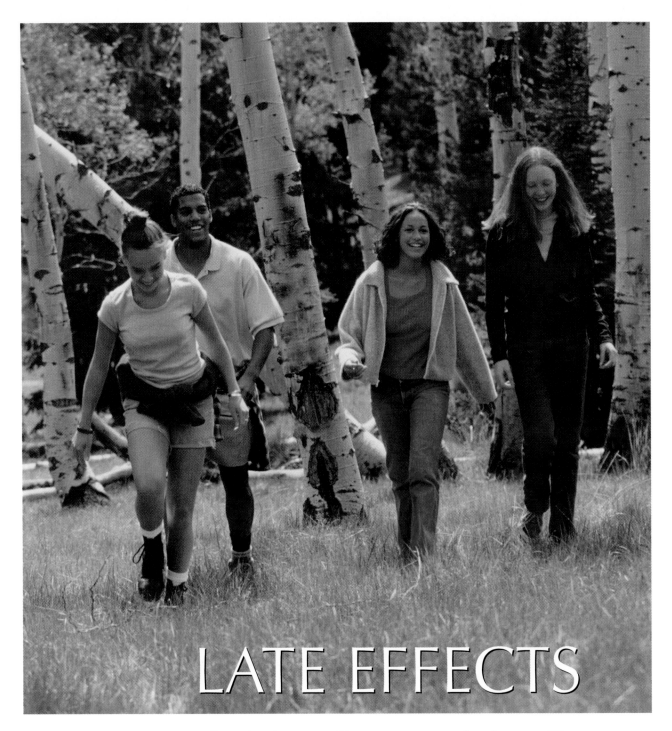

LATE EFFECTS
(OF CANCER AND
ITS TREATMENT)

As THE CHANCE OF CURE CONTINUES TO RISE
FOR CHILDREN WITH CANCER (NOW AT ABOUT 70 PERCENT
FOR ALL TUMORS COMBINED), IT HAS BEEN ESTIMATED
THAT, BY THE YEAR 2010, AS MANY AS ONE IN 250 YOUNG
ADULTS WILL BE A SURVIVOR OF CHILDHOOD CANCER.

This success has been achieved mainly by making the treatment tougher, especially using more drugs in bigger doses. ■ However, this tougher treatment may also cause damage long after it has finished. ■ These effects are being seen more often and may result in serious illness that affects normal functioning.

The risk of developing late effects often increases with time and may not become noticeable until many years after the cancer has been treated. ■ So it is important that your child return regularly for a check-up so that his doctor can detect any problems and treat them early.

Common Late Effects

Growth

Growth problems may be due to surgery or radiation therapy to part of the body involved in growth, such as muscle or bone. ■ Then that part of the body may not grow properly. ■ Reduced overall growth may occur after radiation therapy to the head and neck, which affects hormones involved in growth. ■ Some drugs, such as steroids (like prednisone and dexamethasone), damage bone and muscle, disturbing normal growth. ■ When diagnosed early, growth problems may be corrected.

Learning and Behavior

During treatment, the way your child behaves and how he does at school may be affected. ■ Long-term effects can occur as well, particularly in children who have had brain tumors and in those who have had radiation therapy to the head for other reasons. ■ Some drugs, like methotrexate, can have similar effects, especially when given in high doses. ■ It is important to work with school teachers and others to identify these problems and try to correct them.

The Heart

The muscle of the heart is different from muscles in other parts of the body. ■ It can be damaged easily by certain drugs, particularly those called anthracyclines (including Adriamycin), and by radiation. ■ This damage means that the heart may not grow properly as the child grows. ■ Younger children are affected more often because their hearts are still growing. ■ How much the heart is damaged depends on how much of the drug is used. ■ Testing for early signs of heart damage is done regularly during and after the use of anthracyclines, and the total dose of the drug is limited to reduce the chances of the heart being damaged. ■ Still, heart damage is one of the most common late effects. ■ There are drugs that reduce the normal strain on the heart and may help the heart function better if it has been damaged during cancer treatment. ■ Scientists are looking for alternatives to anthracyclines and for ways to stop these drugs from affecting the heart since they are one of the most powerful treatments for cancer.

Less Common Late Effects

Lungs

Both radiation therapy and certain drugs, including bleomycin and the nitrosoureas BCNU and CCNU, produce inflammation in the lungs that may cause scarring and difficulty in breathing. ■ When possible, the lungs are protected from radiation. ■ Combining radiotherapy to the chest with the above drugs is also avoided. ■ Tests of lung function are done regularly in children who might develop this side effect. ■ Steroids may help children who have developed damage to the lungs.

Kidneys and Bladder

Although these organs can be damaged by radiation, chemotherapy is the more common cause of late effects on kidneys and bladder. ■ Some drugs, like cisplatin and carboplatin, affect kidney function, which may take many months to heal. ■ During this time, your child may have to take extra magnesium by mouth to make up for the unusual amounts lost in the urine. ■ Other drugs, like cyclophosphamide and ifosfamide, can cause long-lasting damage to the bladder. ■ There are no easy ways to treat late effects to the kidneys and bladder, so, whenever possible, they are prevented.

Nerves

Some drugs, like cisplatin, vincristine, and vinblastine, can damage nerves. ■ The common symptoms that occur during treatment usually disappear completely, but some children have long-term problems with weak and wasting muscles, numbness, and tingling sensations. ■ Deafness is a serious late effect as well and may be difficult to pick up in younger children. ■ Regular hearing tests are done in children who receive certain drugs.

Fertility/Reproduction

We don't know much about how cancer treatment affects the ovaries and testes (reproductive organs) of children. ■ It appears that children who have not reached puberty may not develop permanent damage. ■ Later in life, those people who are successful in having children (even if they have difficulty getting and staying pregnant) can be reassured that their children are not at greater risk of illness and other problems than those in the general population.

Second Cancers

Sadly, some children cured of one cancer may develop another cancer as a result of treatment for the first. ■ The most common second cancers are acute myeloid leukemia and sarcomas affecting bone and soft tissues. ■ The chance of developing a second cancer depends on the original cancer and its treatment. ■ Overall, the risk increases with time and is roughly 10 to 20 times greater than in the general population. ■ Second cancers are more likely to develop if a child

- has Hodgkin's disease (especially if he received a drug called procarbazine)
- received high-dose radiation to any part of the body
- was given drugs in the podophyllotoxin family (such as VP16 and VM26).

Every effort is made to avoid or reduce those forms of therapy that can cause second cancers.

As more and more children with cancer are cured with a very low risk of the original cancer returning, we are paying more attention to their quality of life after treatment. ■ Late effects can reduce that quality (and maybe even reduce survival itself). ■ That's why it's important to measure a child's health status during treatment and beyond, in addition to the other things we normally measure such as changes in symptoms, physical examination, blood tests, and x-ray findings. ■ We need to develop ways for the young child, in particular, to report his own state of health. ■ This will allow us to identify and treat problems we wouldn't see otherwise, and it will help improve future treatments that won't cause damaging early and late effects.

CHAPTER 16 IN BRIEF

The day has arrived when your child has completed his cancer treatment. The next challenge is dealing with its possible late effects. Your child's mental, physical, and emotional development may be affected in ways that will pose difficulties later in life. But he can learn to thrive in the face of these difficulties. Regular follow-up clinic visits, which can identify and address problems quickly, are an important part of helping him do this.

Your health care team will have discussed potential late effects when your child was first diagnosed. At that time, these issues may have seemed unimportant; your main concern was curing your child's cancer. Now, at the completion of treatment, take the time to review these possible late effects and discuss your concerns with the team. We share the same goal: helping your child to live a long, happy, and productive life.

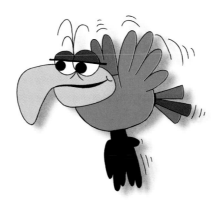

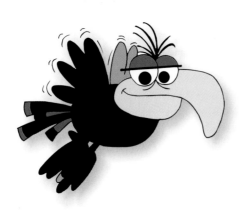

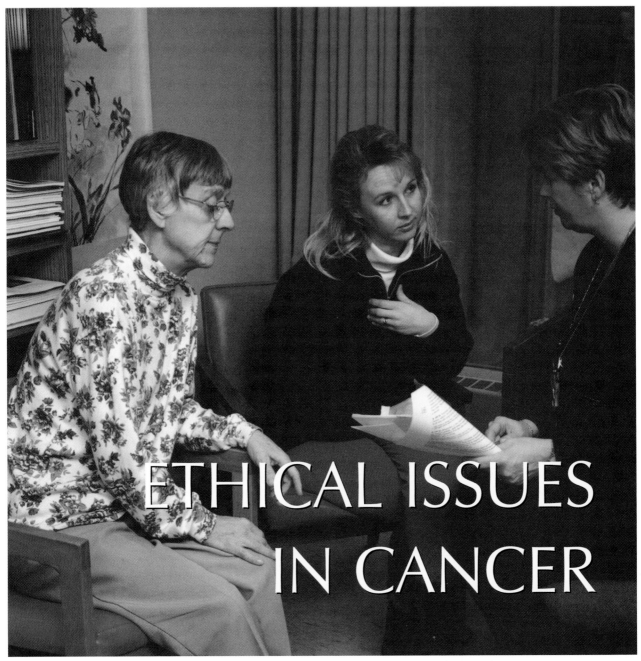

ETHICAL ISSUES
IN CANCER

A DIAGNOSIS OF CANCER PLACES EMOTIONAL, PHYSICAL, AND SPIRITUAL STRAINS UPON YOU AND YOUR CHILD.

Tests and treatments may be very complex, and what is at stake is usually serious, so some of the decisions you have to make can be difficult. ■ Since each family brings different values and feelings to these decisions, they may find themselves in ethical dilemmas when trying to do the right thing.

These dilemmas often arise around
- how open and honest you will be with your child
- your right to reject some forms of treatment
- the demand for treatments not recommended by your child's doctor or the need to continue treatment that doesn't seem to be working
- the role of research in treating your child
- the education and teaching of health professionals.

Openness and Honesty

Over the years, we have learned that the ideal care for your child can be achieved if you, your child, and your child's health care team communicate with and support each other. ■ On the one hand, the clinic staff has to be sensitive to your duties and rights. ■ They have to be honest when telling you about the possible outcome of your child's cancer and be open to the special relationship you have with your child. ■ You, on the other hand, must be aware of the health care team's responsibility to look after your child as well as they can.

Each child has a special insight into his own illness that can help his progress and keep him feeling good about himself. ■ That's why all of us must be honest with children in explaining their cancer in a language they can understand and at a level suited to their age. ■ Children are very sensitive to the changes and emotions that are happening around them during their illness and treatment. ■ By avoiding discussion, your child does not have the chance to talk over his emotions, concerns, and questions. ■ Honesty and a sense of involvement will help your child feel more secure. ■ It will also help him to avoid thoughts that are often more confusing and frightening than the reality.

Health care professionals tend to be more honest and straightforward in explaining what is happening to children than they have been in the past. ■ This may come as a surprise to you, especially if you feel uncomfortable about talking to your child about his illness. ■ It's important to discuss any feelings of discomfort openly with the health care team because you will play a very important part in deciding what they will tell your child.

Consenting to or Rejecting Treatment

Usually, decisions have to be made for children until they reach the age of 16. ■ Each decision must be made with the right information and understanding, including what the treatments involve, what the risks and likely benefits will be, what complications may take place, and whether there are any alternative forms of treatment. ■ Generally, you are expected to make a decision that is in the best interest of your child. ■ You can reject treatment that has not been shown to be effective or stop treatment when it is clearly unsuccessful or when severe side effects occur.

Sometimes, parents don't want their child to have treatment that clinic staff feel is beneficial. ■ It is the legal responsibility of the staff to ensure that the child receives that treatment. ■ There are a number of different ways that a disagreement can be addressed; these are described at the end of this chapter. ■ Similar approaches can be used when a child disagrees with his parents or when parents find themselves disagreeing with each other.

Alternative Treatment

It may be tempting to use alternative therapies. ■ It is frightening to think about losing a child, and there may be pressure from friends or the community to look for new or different therapies, megavitamins, and other non-medical treatments. ■ Unfortunately, these treatments create false hopes, long trips, and financial stress. ■ You can't be denied the right to a second opinion or an alternative course of therapy, but the clinic staff is responsible for ensuring that your child gets the best possible treatment and for avoiding ineffective, dangerous treatments.

Research

At first, children are often placed on standard forms of treatment that have been shown to be useful. ■ However, each child will be treated as an individual, and treatment will be changed to meet his needs.

Despite the large improvements in the treatment of childhood cancer, it will always be true that treatment can get better. ■ Using carefully controlled, safe clinical research is an important part of health care. ■ Research that looks at the causes of cancer and new forms of treatment will help children in the future and may often help a participating child and family now. ■ The use of experimental drugs, treatments, or any other research is watched closely by the government and hospital research committees. ■ Obtaining your consent for research is always necessary, and you can choose not to have your child involved or to withdraw from it later. ■ With the strict regulations now controlling research in children, a research treatment may often be better than a standard therapy.

In research, as well as in standard treatment, you and your child should be involved in making decisions if possible. ■ Generally, children over the age of seven should be aware that a procedure or treatment is part of a research project and should have the opportunity to not take part, withdraw from it, or agree for it to continue. ■ If you or your child withdraws from the research, you can be assured that he will still receive the best care and most effective form of treatment.

Teaching in the Cancer Clinic

Understanding the different kinds of childhood cancer, the drugs used in treating it, and dealing with side effects is complex. ■ It is usually done by experienced health care professionals in a large teaching hospital (a hospital that is connected to a medical school). ■ You and your child will deal with the health care team and many people who are learning, including residents and medical students. ■ Medical students will not normally play a big role in your child's care; they will only watch and do very simple procedures. ■ You and your child have the right to ask that students not be involved in your child's care, but we hope you understand that you and your child are often their most important teachers, even more than lectures or textbooks.

How to Deal with Difficult Problems

The health care team, including the pediatric oncologist, social worker, child life staff, and clinic nurses, can help you come to agreement over a difficult decision. ■ Sometimes, the hospital chaplain may be helpful. ■ Spiritual advisors, ministers, best friends, or family can also help you make the right decisions. ■ Feel free to suggest or request this outside help. ■ Finally, in situations that are especially difficult, hospitals usually have an ethics consultant or ethics committee who can discuss difficult issues. ■ The last step of asking the courts to make a decision is rarely needed.

Cooperation between you and your child's health care professionals can help your child continue to grow physically, emotionally, and spiritually. ■ Fears about your child's illness can be addressed, and, most important, the dignity and humanity of even very sick and dying children can be preserved.

CHAPTER 17 IN BRIEF

When your child has cancer, you and your family will ride a roller coaster of emotions. Talking openly and honestly with your child and his health care team is a meaningful way to "ride out" these emotions. Tell your child the truth about his condition. He will know something is terribly wrong and may think he is dying unless you explain that he has cancer and that its treatment is intended to make him better.

You and your child have rights. Your values and concerns are important, and your health care team will consider them carefully as decisions are made about your child's care. Some decisions will be more difficult and may call for lengthy discussions. Remember that your input is critical to achieving the best outcome for your child.

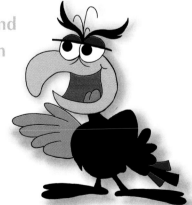

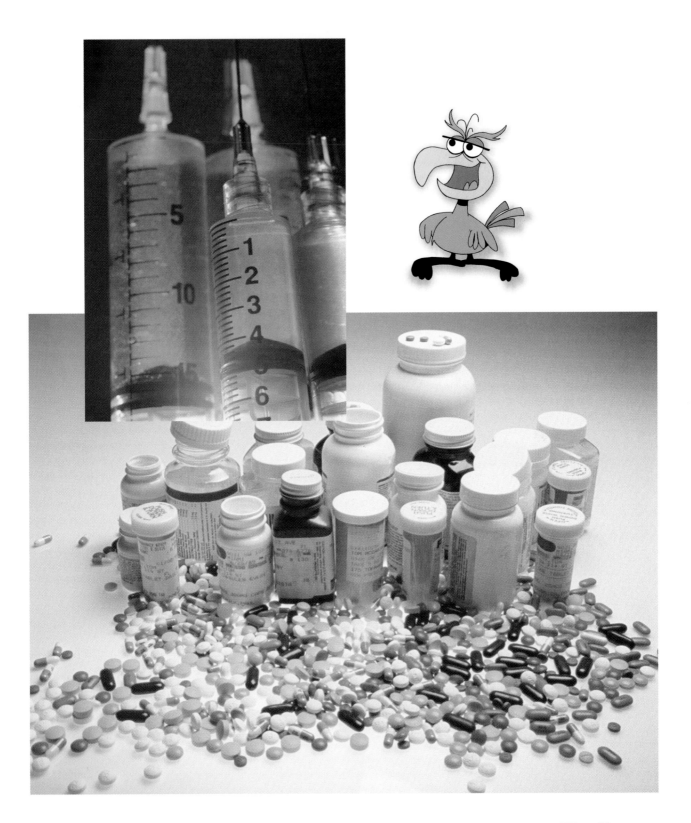

DRUGS

ACETAMINOPHEN (Tylenol, Tempra, Novogesic, Robigesic, others)

Available as an oral liquid, tablets, and suppositories. ■ Used to alleviate fevers and to treat mild pain and discomfort. ■ It is recommended that you always have a supply of this medication at home (and when travelling) to give to your child should a fever develop. ■ The use of acetaminophen (or any other drug) suppositories is not encouraged (especially at times when your child is neutropenic). ■ Inform your physician when a fever develops since this is often the first sign of infection.

Side Effects: Generally, this drug is very well tolerated. ■ Some children may experience some stomach upset with this medication but giving it with some food often alleviates this problem. ■ This drug is eliminated by the liver and may have additive toxic effects to other drugs that may cause liver injury. ■ Note: Do not use aspirin (ASA) or aspirin-containing products to treat your child's fever or discomfort.

ALLOPURINOL (Zyloprim, Novo-Purinol, Apo-Allopurinol, others)

Available as white or pale orange tablets. ■ An injectable (investigational) form is also available. ■ This drug is used to prevent the accumulation of high amounts of uric acid in the bloodstream and attendant risk to the kidneys. ■ Uric acid is a breakdown product of cell turnover/death. ■ It may be elevated at the time of diagnosis and soon after chemotherapy begins. ■ Most children are placed on this drug for a short period of time soon after diagnosis.

Side Effects: Generally well tolerated, but nausea/vomiting, drowsiness, and dizziness are rare side effects. ■ Some children will experience a metallic taste in the mouth while on this drug. Skin rashes do occur more often if your child is also receiving penicillin-type drugs (ampicillin in particular) at the same time. ■ Such rashes do not indicate a penicillin allergy. ■ This drug also interferes with the metabolism of 6-mercaptopurine. ■ If your child is receiving both of these drugs, the dose of 6-mercaptopurine is usually reduced.

AMSACRINE (m-AMSA, AMSA PD)

A clear red/orange liquid that is given by injection* into a vein or central catheter such as a Port-A-Cath or Hickman/Broviac type.

Side Effects: Nausea and vomiting, rashes (usually occur with the first dose or if given near the time of radiation therapy), mouth and gut ulceration, bone marrow suppression, and hair loss may occur. ■ The drug is eliminated partially in the urine and thus may cause some red to orange discoloration. ■ This drug also has cumulative toxicity to the heart. ■ Routine serial tests of heart function (echocardiogram) will be performed to detect any early damage so that the dose of the drug can be modified.

*May cause tissue damage or irritation if it leaks out of a vein.

ASPARAGINASE (Kidrolase, L-asparaginase)

A clear, colorless liquid that must be given by injection into muscle; a so-called IM injection.

Side Effects: Pain at the injection site, tiredness, fevers, possible allergic reactions, which usually show up as a rash but may be accompanied by swelling and/or a drop in blood pressure. ■ This drug can be toxic to the pancreas, resulting in sudden onset of inflammation of this organ with abdominal pain. ■ Blood and urine tests are monitored routinely to check the effects on the pancreas. ■ This drug also affects proteins that the body requires for blood clotting. ■ The imbalance in these proteins may result in your child developing spontaneous blood clots (venous thrombosis or stroke) or bleeding. ■ Nausea and vomiting do not usually occur with asparaginase.

BLEOMYCIN (Blenoxane, Bleo)

A clear, colorless liquid that is given by intravenous injection.

Side Effects: Allergic reactions (fevers, chills, cough, shortness of breath) can occur with this medication. ■ Other side effects include hair loss, skin rashes, and increased pigmentation. ■ This drug can cause cumulative injury to the lungs. ■ This risk is increased if lung irradiation is also required or cannot otherwise be avoided. ■ Your child will have routine serial tests of lung function to detect any early signs of damage and thus permit the dose of the drug to be modified. ■ This drug can also cause mild injury to the liver. ■ Nausea and vomiting and bone marrow suppression do not usually occur with this agent.

BUSULFAN (Busulphan, Myleran)

Small, round white tablets that are taken by mouth.

Side Effects: The principal side effect is bone marrow suppression (maximal 10 to 14 days after taking the drug). ■ Skin rashes may occur. ■ This drug can have significant effects on the reproductive tissues and result in impaired fertility or sterility. ■ It also has cumulative toxic effects on the lungs, which may be additive to other lung-injuring agents. ■ Your child will have routine serial tests of lung function performed to detect any signs of injury early.

CARBOPLATIN (Paraplatin, Paraplatin AQ)

A clear, colorless liquid that is given by intravenous injection.

Side Effects: Nausea and vomiting are common with this medication and vary with the dose of the drug. ■ The drug leaches into saliva and thus can affect your child's appetite and sense of taste. ■ Bone marrow depression is common and occurs 14 to 21 days after the drug is given. ■ This drug can be toxic to the kidneys and the ears but slightly less so than cisplatin. ■ Your child will receive vigorous hydration with intravenous fluids to minimize the potential for toxicity. ■ The drug commonly causes a temporary inability on the part of the kidney to conserve magnesium. ■ Your child may be required to take a magnesium supplement while on chemotherapy and for some time after completion of chemotherapy. ■ Tests of kidney and hearing function are performed routinely to detect any damage.

CARMUSTINE (BCNU, BiCNU)

A clear, straw-colored liquid given by intravenous injection.*

Side Effects: Nausea and vomiting are quite common. ■ Bone marrow depression occurs but usually three to five weeks after a dose. ■ This drug may cause lung injury or add to the injury caused by other lung toxic drugs. ■ Routine serial tests will be performed to monitor lung function.

*May cause tissue damage or irritation if it leaks out of the vein.

CHLORPROMAZINE (Largactil)

Available as white or light beige oral tablets, a clear or yellow-colored oral solution, or as a clear, straw-colored injectable liquid. ■ This drug is used to alleviate nausea/vomiting associated with chemotherapy and occasionally in sedative "cocktails" prior to certain procedures such as lumbar punctures or bone marrow aspiration/biopsy.

Side Effects: Drowsiness, dry mouth, nasal congestion, and increased heart rate are most commonly encountered. ■ This drug may also cause extra-pyramidal reactions, which manifest as sudden-onset muscle rigidity/spasm. ■ These are treated with diphenhydramine and sometimes benztropine. ■ This drug may make your child's skin more sensitive to sunlight, so it is recommended that he wear a good sunscreen (SPF 30 or higher) while outdoors. ■ A rare side effect in children is a sudden drop in blood pressure upon standing from a sitting or lying position (orthostatic hypotension), which may result in dizziness and/or fainting. ■ This drug may also decrease the seizure threshold in children prone to seizures.

CISPLATIN (Platinol, Cisplatinum, CDDP)

A clear, colorless liquid that is given by intravenous injection.

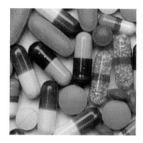

Side Effects: The side effects of this medication are virtually identical to those of carboplatin (see above), except that nausea and vomiting are usually more severe and the risk of kidney and hearing toxicity is slightly greater.

CLADRIBINE (CdA, 2CdA, Leustatin)

A clear, colorless liquid that is given by intravenous injection usually as a continuous infusion.

Side Effects: Nausea and vomiting may occur but are usually quite mild. ■ Bone marrow depression (maximal at two to three weeks after receiving the drug) is to be expected.

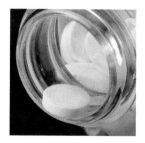

COTRIMOXAZOLE (Septra, Bactrim, Apo-Sulfatrim, Novo-Trimel, others)

Available in round (regular-strength) or oval (double-strength) tablets, as a pink oral suspension, and in an intravenous form. ■ This is a combination antibiotic composed of a sulfa drug and a drug called trimethoprim. ■ This agent is often used to treat a variety of childhood infections. ■ This drug is also very effective in treating pneumonias caused by an organism called *Pneumocystis carinii*. ■ Children with certain types of cancer or on certain types of chemotherapy programs have a higher risk of developing this type of pneumonia. ■ If your child falls into this category, he will be placed on a routine schedule of cotrimoxazole prophylaxis in which this drug is administered in a low dose (three days per week) to prevent the development of this type of pneumonia.

Side Effects: This drug is generally well tolerated and can be given with food or on an empty stomach. ■ This medication can increase the sensitivity of your child's skin to sunlight; therefore, a strong sunscreen (SPF 30) should be worn by your child when exposed to the sun. ■ Skin rashes can occur with this medication and are usually indicative of an allergy to

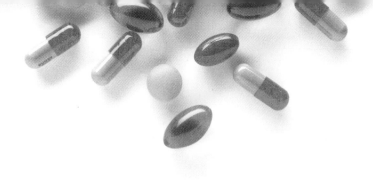

the sulfa component. ■ The trimethoprim component may cause bone marrow suppression in addition to other drugs your child is receiving. ■ Inform the physician if you know that your child is allergic to sulfa-type drugs so that an alternative agent (for example, pentamidine) may be prescribed.

CYCLOPHOSPHAMIDE (Procytox, Cyclo, Cytoxan)

A clear, colorless liquid that is given by intravenous injection. ■ This drug is also available in tablet form, but this form is rarely used in children.

Side Effects: Nausea and vomiting occur and are related to the dose of the drug administered. ■ Hair loss and bone marrow depression (maximal seven to 14 days after receiving the drug) are common. ■ Mouth sores (ulcerations) may occur. ■ This drug is metabolized extensively by the liver, and these metabolites are excreted in the urine. ■ Some of these metabolites are toxic to the bladder wall and can cause irritation and inflammation. ■ Your child will have his urine checked regularly to look for any early signs of damage. ■ The use of lots of intravenous fluids (to dilute these toxins) and encouraging your child to empty his bladder often are useful measures in preventing this type of injury. ■ On occasion, when high doses of this drug must be given, an additional agent called MESNA is utilized. ■ This drug passes into the urine and binds with the toxic metabolites of cyclophosphamide to prevent bladder injury. ■ Cyclophosphamide also has significant toxic effects on the reproductive system and may contribute to the formation of second cancers.

CYTARABINE (Cytosine Arabinoside, Cytosar, Ara-C)

A clear, colorless liquid that is given as an injection intravenously or occasionally subcutaneously. ■ This is one of several medications that is sometimes instilled into the spinal fluid.

Side Effects: Nausea and vomiting occur and are related to the dose of the drug. ■ Bone marrow depression (maximal 10 to 14 days after receiving the drug), mouth and gut ulceration, diarrhea, and hair loss are all very common side effects. ■ This drug also occasionally causes fevers.

DACARBAZINE (DTIC)

A clear, pale, straw-colored to colorless liquid that is given by intravenous injection.*

Side Effects: Nausea and vomiting are common and usually severe. ■ A metallic taste in the mouth is common and may affect your child's appetite. ■ Bone marrow depression (maximal 10 to 14 days after receiving the drug) and pain along the vein used for injection may occur as well as a flu-like syndrome of fever, headache, and malaise. ■ This drug also has toxic effects on the reproductive system and may result in impaired fertility or sterility.

*May cause tissue irritation or damage if it leaks out of the vein.

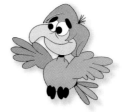

DACTINOMYCIN (Cosmegen, Lyovac, Actinomycin D)

A clear yellow liquid given as an injection intravenously.*

Side Effects: Nausea and vomiting, mouth and gut ulcers, diarrhea, and hair loss are all common side effects. ■ Bone marrow suppression occurs and is maximal 10 to 14 days after receiving the drug. ■ Hair loss and skin rashes may occur. ■ These rashes are common if your child receives radiation therapy soon after a dose of this medication.

*May cause tissue irritation or damage if it leaks out of the vein.

DAUNORUBICIN (Daunomycin, Cerubidine)

A clear red liquid that is given by intravenous injection.*

Side Effects: Nausea and vomiting occur and are related to the dose of the drug given. ■ Bone marrow suppression (maximal 10 to 14 days after receiving the drug) is usual. ■ Mouth sores (ulcerations) and diarrhea may occur. ■ The drug is excreted in part via the kidneys in the urine, and some red-orange discoloration of the urine may occur. ■ In cumulative amounts, this drug can be toxic to the heart. ■ Your child will have routine serial tests (echocardiogram) of heart function to look for any early signs of damage.

*May cause tissue irritation and damage if it leaks out of the vein.

DEXAMETHASONE (Decadron)

Small oval pale white or green tablets that are taken by mouth. ■ Also available as a clear, colorless liquid that may be injected intravenously.

Side Effects: The most notable side effects of this medication include bone mineral loss resulting in bony aches and pains and alterations in mood and behavior of the child. ■ Other side effects include changes in fat and sugar metabolism leading to a temporary diabetic state and stimulation of the appetite. ■ When taken orally, this medication can cause stomach upset. ■ Taking the medication with meals often alleviates this. ■ When given in slightly higher than usual doses, this drug is an excellent anti-emetic (anti-nauseant) medication.

DIMENHYDRINATE (Gravol, Travamine, Novo-dimenate, others)

Available as a clear, colorless liquid for injection, peach-colored oral tablets, a clear yellow oral solution, and as blue/white sustained-release capsules. ■ Suppositories are also available. ■ This drug is used to alleviate nausea/vomiting.

Side Effects: Drowsiness, blurred vision, dizziness, and dryness of the mouth are most frequently encountered. ■ Dimenhydrinate is an antihistamine-type drug and may cause paradoxical central nervous system stimulation in some children. ■ This drug may also decrease the seizure threshold in children prone to seizures.

DIPHENHYDRAMINE (Benadryl, others)

An antihistamine that is available as a clear, colorless liquid for injection, pink/white or pink/clear oral capsules, and as a clear red oral solution. ■ This drug is often used to alleviate allergic reactions (e.g., hives) to transfusions or to other medications. ■ This agent is often given together with some anti-nauseant medications such as chlorpromazine, metoclopramide, and prochlorperazine to reduce the risk of extra-pyramidal reactions associated with these drugs.

Side Effects: Drowsiness, dizziness, dry mouth, and blurred vision. ■ As with dimenhydrinate, antihistamines can cause paradoxical central nervous system stimulation in some children. ■ This drug may also lower the seizure threshold in children prone to seizures.

DOXORUBICIN (Adriamycin)

A clear red/orange liquid given by intravenous injection.*

Side Effects: Nausea and vomiting are common and dose dependent. ■ Bone marrow suppression occurs and is maximal 10 to 14 days after receiving the drug. ■ Mouth ulceration and diarrhea may occur. ■ Hair loss is common. ■ A skin rash may develop if your child receives radiation therapy soon after receiving doxorubicin. ■ The drug, like a number of others, is toxic to the heart. ■ This toxicity occurs with cumulative doses beyond which the risk of heart toxicity rises significantly. ■ Your child will have routine serial tests (echocardiogram) to monitor heart function. ■ This drug is also partially excreted in the urine; thus, some red/orange discoloration of the urine may occur.

*May cause tissue irritation and damage if it leaks out of the vein.

EMLA CREAM

A white cream that is a mixture of two local anesthetics. ■ When applied to the skin and left on for 45 to 60 minutes, the cream anesthetizes the skin; thus, insertion of a needle through this area of the skin (to start an IV, for a lumbar puncture, or to access a Port-A-Cath) can be accomplished in a painless manner.

Side Effects: Essentially none since virtually no drug is absorbed. ■ Your child may, however, develop a local skin reaction (redness, itching) if he is allergic to either anesthetic in the cream, although this is very rare. ■ The cream is available without a prescription from your pharmacist.

ETOPOSIDE (Vepesid, VP16)

A clear, straw-colored liquid that is first diluted and then injected intravenously.*

Side Effects: Nausea and vomiting may occur but are usually mild. ■ Hair loss is common. Mouth sores (ulcerations) may occur. ■ Allergic reactions may occur, as well as changes in blood pressure during administration of this drug. ■ Your child will have his blood pressure monitored closely during and for some time after the infusion is complete. ■ Depending on the dose and schedule of administration of this drug, it may predispose to the development of secondary cancers (leukemias).

*May cause tissue irritation and damage if it leaks out of the vein.

FILGRASTIM (G-CSF, Neupogen)

Available as a clear, colorless liquid for subcutaneous (and occasionally intravenous) injection. ■ This is a hormone-type drug that is administered after chemotherapy to stimulate the bone marrow to produce neutrophils and thus reduce the degree of neutropenia and risk of infection with certain chemotherapy regimens given for certain types of cancer. ■ This drug is not available for routine use in some jurisdictions. ■ Your physician/nurse/pharmacist will be able to answer any questions you have regarding the use of this drug for your child.

Side Effects: The most frequently encountered side effects are bony aches and pains and occasional low-grade fevers. ■ These respond very well to acetaminophen (Tylenol). ■ There may also be some minor discomfort from the injection.

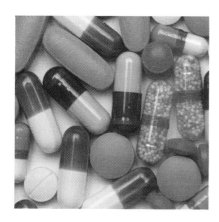

FOLINIC ACID (Leucovorin, Citrovorum Factor)

Available as a clear to straw-colored solution for injection and as white oral tablets. ■ This drug is a vitamin and is used in chemotherapy protocols that use moderate to high-dose methotrexate. ■ The purpose of this drug is to by-pass the toxic effect of methotrexate and prevent excessive toxicity. ■ The dose and schedule (timing) of this drug will vary from program to program but must be followed precisely to prevent undue toxicity.

Side Effects: Nausea and vomiting are rare and can be alleviated by taking the drug with some food. ■ Skin rashes are very rare. ■ Note: Do not confuse folinic acid with folic acid.

HYDROXYUREA (Hydrea)

Large bright pink and green capsules that are taken by mouth. ■ For small children, the capsules may be opened gently and the contents placed in a small amount of food for ease of administration. ■ Wash your hands promptly after handling opened capsules.

Side Effects: Nausea and vomiting are usually mild. ■ Hair loss is uncommon. ■ Bone marrow suppression occurs and is maximal 14 to 20 days after taking the medication. ■ Diarrhea or constipation may occur but are rare. ■ There may be changes in skin color and nails. ■ Rashes may occur, especially if your child receives radiation therapy soon after the time of taking this drug.

IFOSFAMIDE (Iphosphamide, Holoxan, Ifex)

A clear, colorless liquid given by intravenous injection.

Side Effects: Nausea and vomiting are very common and are dose related. ■ Mouth sores (ulcerations) and diarrhea are quite common. ■ Bone marrow suppression occurs and is maximal seven to 14 days after the drug is given. ■ Hair loss is common. ■ This drug, like cyclophosphamide, is also metabolized extensively and excreted by the kidneys in the urine. ■ These metabolites can cause significant irritation and inflammation of the bladder wall, which may result in pain on urination or passing of blood in the urine. ■ This appears to be a greater risk with ifosfamide than with cyclophosphamide. ■ Therefore, in addition to vigorous hydration with intravenous fluids and encouraging your child to empty his bladder often, MESNA (a drug that binds these toxins in the bladder) is used routinely. ■ Your child will have his urine checked routinely to determine if there is any evidence of inflammation or irritation of the bladder. ■ Like cyclophosphamide, ifosfamide also has significant toxicity to the reproductive system and may be associated with the development of second cancers.

LOMUSTINE (CCNU, CeeNU)

Capsules that may be purple, purple/green, or green in color depending on strength. ■ These are taken by mouth. ■ In small children, the capsules may be opened and the contents sprinkled on some food to facilitate administration. ■ Do not mix the contents of the capsules with juices or milk. ■ Wash your hands promptly after handling.

Side Effects: Nausea and vomiting are common but can be alleviated somewhat by giving the medication at bedtime. ■ Hair loss is rare. ■ Bone marrow suppression occurs but may not be evident for three to eight weeks. ■ The drug can have toxic effects on the liver, may cause lung injury, or may add to the injury caused by other lung toxic drugs. ■ Routine blood tests will be performed to monitor liver function, and routine serial tests will be performed to assess lung function. ■ This drug will have toxic effects on the reproductive organs and may cause impaired fertility or sterility.

MECHLORETHAMINE (Nitrogen Mustard, Mustargen)

A clear, colorless liquid given by intravenous injection.*

Side Effects: Nausea and vomiting are common and usually severe. ■ This drug may give your child a metallic taste in the mouth and thus affect his appetite. ■ Hair loss and diarrhea may occur. ■ Bone marrow suppression occurs and is maximal 14 to 21 days after receiving the drug. ■ This drug will have toxic effects on the reproductive organs and may result in impaired fertility or sterility.

*May cause tissue irritation and damage if it leaks out of the vein.

MERCAPTOPURINE (6-MP, Purinethol)

Round, scored, white tablets that are taken by mouth. ■ You may be required to split the tablets into halves or quarters in order to give the correct dose. ■ Wash your hands promptly after handling. ■ This medication is absorbed better when given on an empty stomach at bedtime with some clear fluids. ■ Do not give with milk.

Side Effects: Nausea and vomiting are uncommon with this medication. ■ Bone marrow suppression occurs and is maximal approximately 14 days after beginning a course of therapy. ■ Hair loss is uncommon. ■ This drug may cause mild injury to the liver. ■ Your child will have blood tests routinely to monitor liver function. ■ Rashes can occur with mercaptopurine.

MESNA (Uromitexan)

A clear, colorless liquid for injection, this liquid may also be used orally. ■ This agent is routinely given with ifosfamide and in certain situations with cyclophosphamide. ■ This drug (along with vigorous hydration) is used to protect the bladder from harmful by-products (metabolites) of ifosfamide and cyclophosphamide.

Side Effects: Nausea and vomiting may occur if the drug is injected too rapidly;

otherwise, no other side effects are noted. ■ Note: If your child is receiving ifosfamide or cyclophosphamide, encourage him to empty his bladder often.

METHOTREXATE (Amethopterin, MTX)

A clear, yellow solution that can be injected intravenously or intramuscularly and on occasion is given into the spinal fluid (intrathecally). ■ This drug is also available as small yellow tablets that can be taken by mouth. ■ However, since the absorption of oral methotrexate is very variable, the injectable route is preferred. ■

Side Effects: Nausea and vomiting are uncommon at low doses of this drug but can be significant at very high doses. ■ Mouth and gut ulceration and diarrhea may occur but are more common when high doses are used. ■ This drug has toxic effects on the liver; thus, your child will have routine blood tests performed to assess liver function. ■ The dose of this drug may have to be reduced if significant impairment of liver function occurs. ■ When very high doses are given, the drug can be toxic to the kidneys, due to precipitation (crystallization) in the presence of acidic urine. ■ Thus, children getting high doses of methotrexate will routinely be given extra IV fluid hydration and have their urine alkalinized with sodium bicarbonate (given intravenously). ■ As well, in this circumstance, an additional drug called folinic acid (leucovorin) is given to reverse the toxic effects of high-dose methotrexate. ■ Hair loss is uncommon. ■ This drug can also sensitize the skin to sunlight. ■ It is therefore highly recommended that your child wear a strong (SPF 30) sunscreen when exposed to the sun.

METOCLOPRAMIDE (Maxeran, Reglan)

A vailable as white or pale blue oral tablets, a clear, colorless oral solution, and as a clear, colorless solution for injection. ■ This drug is a very effective agent in controlling the nausea and vomiting associated with cancer chemotherapy.

Side Effects: Drowsiness and dizziness are most common; abdominal cramps occur occasionally, as does diarrhea. ■ Rarely, extra-pyramidal reactions (muscle spasm/rigidity) can occur, but the administration of diphenhydramine (Benadryl) together with metoclopramide reduces this risk. ■ This drug may decrease the seizure threshold in children prone to seizures.

MITOXANTRONE (Novantrone)

A clear, deep blue liquid that is given by intravenous injection.

Side Effects: Nausea and vomiting occur but are usually mild to moderate. ■ Mouth sores may occur with certain administration schedules. ■ This drug, like others (doxorubicin, daunorubicin, amsacrine), does have toxic effects on the heart. ■ Your child will have routine serial tests (echocardiogram) of heart function performed to detect any early damage and thus permit modification of the dose of this medication. ■ The drug may cause liver injury. ■ Your child will have routine tests of liver function performed. ■ Hair loss is common. ■ Bone marrow suppression occurs and is maximal 10 to 14 days after receiving the drug. ■ Skin rashes are rare but can occur if your child receives radiation therapy soon after receiving mitoxantrone. ■ This drug may have significant toxic effects on the reproductive organs and result in impaired fertility or sterility. ■ The drug is eliminated in part by the kidneys through the urine. ■ Some blue/green discoloration of the urine may be observed.

NABILONE (Cesamet)

Available only as blue/white capsules for oral ingestion. ■ This drug is a highly effective anti-nauseant that is derived from THC, the active ingredient in marijuana. ■ Although very effective, side effects limit the usefulness of this agent.

Side Effects: Drowsiness, dizziness, ataxia (stumbling gait), euphoria/dysphoria (an unpleasant "high"), depersonalization (out-of-body experiences), dry mouth, blurred vision, and rapid heartbeat are all commonly encountered side effects with this drug.

ONDANSETRON (Zofran)

Available as yellow oval tablets for oral use or as a clear, colorless liquid for injection. ■ This drug is the most potent and most effective anti-nauseant medication for controlling severe nausea and vomiting that occurs with the use of certain anti-cancer drugs (e.g., high doses of cisplatinum) or with some types of radiation therapy. ■ Your child may or may not require the use of this drug depending on the type of chemotherapy he receives and how he tolerates therapy.

Side Effects: Generally well tolerated, with headache being the most common side effect. Other rare side effects are dizziness, constipation, and diarrhea.

PACLITAXEL (Taxol)

A clear, colorless liquid that is given by intravenous injection,* usually as a continuous infusion over several hours.

Side Effects: Nausea and vomiting are common. ■ Muscle and joint pain occur frequently. ■ The use of acetaminophen (Tylenol) may provide some symptomatic relief. ■ This drug also causes toxicity to nerves, which usually occurs as a burning or tingling sensation in the hands (especially fingers) and feet. ■ This toxicity appears to be cumulative in nature and may be partially or completely reversible. ■ Allergic reactions to this drug are common; thus, children are usually pre-medicated with an antihistamine and/or steroid drug to minimize such reactions. ■ Hair loss is common. ■ This drug may cause mild liver injury. ■ Your child will have blood tests performed routinely to assess liver function. ■ Changes in heart rate and blood pressure are common during the infusion of this drug. ■ Your child will have his heart rate and blood pressure monitored closely during each infusion and for some time after it is completed.

*May cause tissue irritation and damage if it leaks out of the vein.

PENTAMIDINE (Pentacarinat, Pneumopent, others)

A clear, colorless solution that can be administered intravenously (IV), intramuscularly (IM), or by inhalation. ■ Children who are allergic to cotrimoxazole and require prophylaxis for *Pneumocystis carinii* pneumonia may receive pentamidine by inhalation approximately once per month. ■ Side effects with this mode of administration (as distinct from IV or IM administration) are limited to mild shortness of breath or a feeling of tightness in the chest (bronchospasm) in children whose airways are particularly reactive (e.g., children with asthma).

Side Effects: (with IV/IM administration) Nausea, occasionally fevers, and discomfort at the injection site have been reported in response to receiving this drug by IV or IM injection. ■ This drug can also cause sudden large drops in blood pressure; therefore, your child will have frequent blood pressure determinations done while on this drug. ■ This drug can cause injury to the kidneys, liver, and pancreas. ■ In particular, injury to the pancreas can result in changes in blood sugar levels. ■ Thus, routine blood tests will be performed to monitor for injury to these organs and to check blood sugar levels. ■ Bone marrow suppression and skin rashes can occur but are uncommon. ■ Disturbances in heart rhythm have also been reported but are very rare.

PREDNISONE (Pred)

Small, white, scored tablets that are taken by mouth. ■ This medication may be prepared in a liquid suspension for small infants and children. ■ This drug may cause stomach upset and therefore should be given with food.

Side Effects: Increased appetite and weight gain are common. ■ This drug can cause changes in fat and sugar metabolism and may result in a temporary diabetic state. ■ The drug also causes loss of mineral from bones, so your child may experience bony aches and pains while taking this medication. ■ Some children may limp when they try to walk due to the bony discomfort. ■ Changes in mood are very common.

PROCARBAZINE (Natulan)

Small white capsules that are taken by mouth.

Side Effects: Nausea and vomiting are common. ■ Dryness of the mouth, diarrhea, or constipation may occur. ■ Bone marrow suppression occurs but may not be evident for two to four weeks. ■ Skin rashes can occur, particularly if your child receives radiation therapy soon after a course of oral procarbazine. ■ Procarbazine may interact with a number of foods and drugs. ■ The following should be avoided: aged cheeses (Camembert, Emmenthal); beer and wine (especially red wine, such as Chianti); caffeine-containing foods and drinks such as coffee, tea, and chocolate; aged meats such as salami, bologna, summer sausage, smoked or pickled meat or fish, overripe fruits, bananas, fava beans, and soy sauce. ■ Any over-the-counter cough and cold preparations containing phenylpropanolamine, such as Neo-Citran, Dristan, and others, should be avoided. ■ If in doubt, ask the pharmacist. ■ It is advisable to avoid these while on and for two weeks after taking procarbazine.

PROCHLORPERAZINE (Stemetil, Compazine)

Available as peach-colored tablets, a clear red oral solution, and as a clear, straw-colored liquid for injection. ■ This drug is effective in alleviating the nausea and vomiting associated with certain chemotherapy.

Side Effects: Drowsiness, dizziness, dry mouth, rapid heart beat, and nasal congestion are commonly encountered with the use of this drug. ■ This drug, like chlorpromazine and metoclopramide, may cause extra-pyramidal-type reactions. ■ The use of diphenhydramine (Benadryl), together with this drug, reduces the risk of such reactions occurring. ■ This drug may make your child's skin more sensitive to sunlight, so ensure that he wears a good sunscreen (SPF 30 or higher) if spending time outdoors. ■ Very rarely, children may experience a drop in blood pressure when standing up from a sitting or lying position; this may result in dizziness or fainting. ■ This drug may also lower the seizure threshold in children prone to seizures.

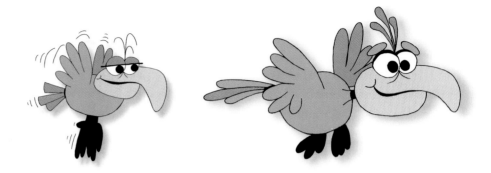

TENIPOSIDE (Vumon, VM26)

A clear, straw-colored liquid that is diluted and then injected intravenously.*

Side Effects: Nausea and vomiting occur but are usually mild. ■ Changes in blood pressure during the infusion and allergic reactions may occur. ■ Your child will have his blood pressure monitored throughout the infusion and for some time after. ■ Bone marrow suppression occurs and is maximal eight to 10 days after receiving the drug. ■ This drug may cause fevers. ■ These usually respond to acetaminophen (Tylenol). ■ However, all fevers should be reported to the physician. ■ This drug may also increase the risk of developing second cancers, depending on the dose and schedule of administration.

*May cause tissue irritation and damage if it leaks out of the vein.

VINBLASTINE (Velban)

A clear, colorless liquid that is given by intravenous injection.*

Side Effects: Hair loss occurs commonly. ■ Nausea and vomiting are rare. ■ This drug may have mild toxic effects on the liver. ■ Your child will have routine blood tests to monitor liver function. ■ This drug is toxic to the nerves. ■ It usually appears as a tingling or burning sensation in the hands and feet, and you may find your child to be somewhat clumsy. This toxicity may be reversible often over a long time. ■ Occasionally, jaw pain may be experienced. ■ Constipation may occur and result in abdominal discomfort. Bone marrow suppression is common.

*May cause tissue irritation and damage if it leaks out of the vein.

VINCRISTINE (VCR, Oncovin)

A clear, colorless liquid that is given by intravenous injection.*

Side Effects: The side-effect profile of vincristine is very similar to that of vinblastine (see above), except for bone marrow suppression. ■ This drug can be toxic to nerves, resulting in a tingling or burning sensation of the hands and feet. Jaw pain may occur occasionally, as can constipation. ■ Hair loss is common. ■ This drug may have mild toxic effects on the liver. ■ Your child will have routine blood tests performed to assess liver function.

*May cause tissue irritation and damage if it leaks out of the vein.

NOTES

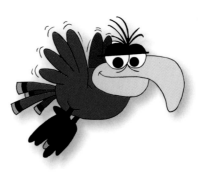

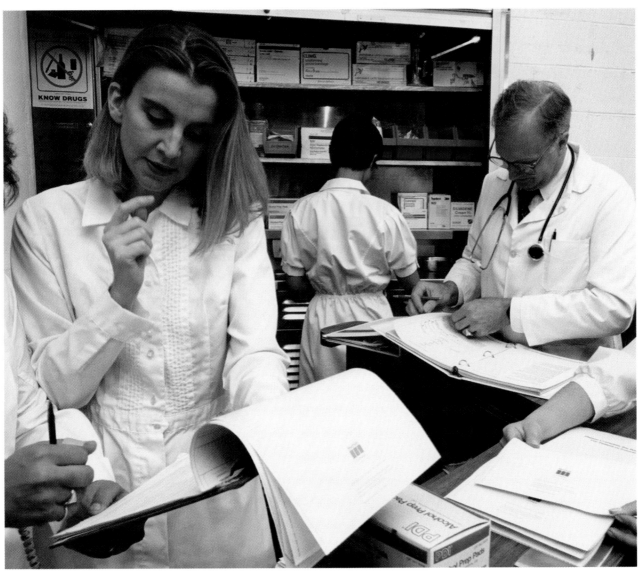

APPENDIX

Acupuncture Piercing of the skin with needles to relieve discomfort.

Agglutination Formation of clumps (e.g., of cells) in a liquid.

Allogeneic Of the same species but different (e.g., a brother or sister).

Alopecia Loss of hair.

Amputation Removal of a limb.

Amylase A protein, produced mainly by the pancreas. Levels of this protein rise in blood and urine when the pancreas is damaged.

Analgesic Relieves pain.

Anemia Below-normal levels of hemoglobin in the blood.

Anesthetic Removing sensation by medication, either in a limited area of the body (local or regional) or generally.

Angiography X-ray examination of blood vessels that are injected with a contrast medium.

Anthracyclines Class of anti-cancer drugs including Adriamycin and Daunomycin.

Antibiotic A medication used to kill or limit the growth of bacterial micro-organisms that cause infection.

Antibody Blood protein that sticks to substances (antigens) that are seen as foreign by the body.

Antiemetic Prevents or reduces nausea and vomiting.

Antihistamine Drug that prevents or reduces allergic reactions.

Anus External opening of the rectum.

Appendectomy Removal of the appendix, an unnecessary small part of the bowel.

Aspiration Removal by suction.

Audiometry Test of hearing.

Autologous Of oneself (e.g., a skin graft from one part of the body to another).

Biopsy Removal of a small part of the living body to make a precise diagnosis.

Bone Marrow Jelly-like material in the center of bones, where blood cells are made.

Carcinogen Agent causing cancer.

Cardiologist Physician trained to diagnose and treat heart disease.

Catheter Flexible tube for gaining access to the circulation or body cavities (e.g., the bladder).

CBC Complete blood count.

Chemotherapy Treatment using drugs.

Chromosomes Structures in the nucleus of a cell, containing DNA (which carries inherited information from parents).

Coagulation Clotting of the blood.

Colon Lower part of the bowel ending in the rectum.

Contrast Medium Liquid used in x-ray examinations that improves the distinction of one structure from another.

Crossmatching Determining whether blood from the donor is compatible with that from the patient, in preparation for transfusion.

CT Scan Computerized tomography; an x-ray examination involving the use of multiple images.

Cystitis Inflammation of the bladder.

Cytochemistry Identification and localization of the chemical parts of the cell.

Cytogenetics Study of the chromosomes.

Cytology Microscopic examination of cells.

Cytopenia Below-normal levels of cells in the blood.

Dermatologist Physician trained to diagnose and treat skin disease.

Diagnosis A statement of the nature of a patient's illness.

Differential Leukocyte Count Proportion of the total white blood cell count composed of each separate cell type (e.g., neutrophils and lymphocytes).

Digestive Tract The entire gut from the mouth to the anus.

DNA Chemical substance carrying inherited information.

Duodenum The part of the digestive tract into which the stomach empties.

Erythrocyte Red blood cell.

Esophagus The "food pipe" that connects the mouth to the stomach.

ESR Erythrocyte sedimentation rate; a blood test often used to look at disease activity.

Febrile Having a temperature above normal.

Ferritin A protein that stores iron.

Granulocyte Type of white blood cell that can digest micro-organisms.

Gynecologist Physician trained to diagnose and treat diseases of the female genital tract.

Hematology Study of the blood and bone marrow.

Hemoglobin Red pigment (contained in erythrocytes) that carries oxygen in the blood.

Hepatitis Inflammation of the liver.

Hives Itchy welts on the skin.

Holistic Considering the patient as a whole—mind, body, and spirit.

Hormone Chemical substance produced in the body that has a specific effect on a certain organ.

Iliac Relating to a hip bone.

Immunity Security system in the body that protects against disease.

Immunology Study of immunity.

Inferior Vena Cavagram Angiography of the main vein that drains blood from the lower half of the body.

Intestinal Obstruction Blockage of the lower part of the digestive tract.

Intrathecal Within the spinal fluid.

Laparotomy A type of small surgical cut in the abdomen.

LDH Lactate dehydrogenase; a protein that is produced by many cells including cancer cells in Ewing's sarcoma and malignant lymphoma.

Leukocyte White blood cell.

Leukopenia Below-normal levels of leukocytes in the blood.

LFT Liver function tests that are performed on a blood sample.

Lymph Gland A dense collection of lymphocytes.

Lymphatic System Nodes and channels that carry lymphocytes outside the blood.

Lymphocyte Type of white blood cell that participates in immunity, especially by producing antibodies and controlling viral infection.

Lymphoma Malignant growth of lymphocytes.

Malignant Relating to cancer.

Metastasis Spread of cancer from one part of the body to another distant part.

MIBG Metaiodobenzylguanidine; an agent that attaches to neuroblastoma cells. As a result, it can be used to search for these cells in the patient after it is injected in a radioactive form.

Micro-organisms Agents, invisible to the naked eye, that are the cause of infections.

MIPS/MEPS Maximal inspiratory pressures and maximal expiratory pressures; measuring the strength of breathing muscles.

Monocyte Type of white blood cells that can digest micro-organisms.

Morbidity Illness.

Mortality Death.

MRI Magnetic resonance imaging; a form of radiologic examination.

Mucosa Lining of hollow organs (e.g., mouth, stomach, bladder, etc).

Nebulizer Device for delivering a spray into the mouth.

Neutropenia Below-normal levels of neutrophils in the blood.

Neutrophil The most common form of granulocyte (type of white blood cells). Others are called eosinophils and basophils.

Node Normal small collection of lymphocytes (type of white blood cells) that becomes swollen in certain cases (e.g., infection).

Nucleus Part of a cell that contains the chromosomes.

Oncology Study of cancer (malignant diseases).

Ovariopexy Elevating and fixing an ovary to the inside of the front wall of the abdomen. This is often done to protect the ovary from receiving radiation during radiotherapy.

Oximetry Measurement of the oxygen content of blood.

Palliative Providing relief but not a cure.

Pancreas Large organ that is deep in the abdomen, behind the stomach. It produces juices that enter the digestive tract and insulin that enters the blood.

Parenteral Not through the digestive tract but by injection (e.g., into a muscle, into a vein).

Petechiae Pin-point purple spots caused by bleeding into the skin.

Phenotyping Determining the surface characteristics of a cell.

Pheresis Separation of parts that make up something (e.g., by centrifugation [spinning]).

Platelet Small particle in the blood that helps prevent bleeding.

Premedication Giving drugs before a test or treatment.

Primitive Not fully developed.

Red Blood Cell A cell that has no nucleus (no chromosomes) and is full of hemoglobin.

Relapse Return of disease.

Remission Disappearance (not a cure) of detectable disease.

Respirology Study of breathing.

Retina Layer at the back of the eye that is sensitive to light. It is connected to the brain by the optic nerve.

Retroperitoneal Behind the back wall of the abdomen.

Scoliosis Curving of the bony spine (vertebrae) to the side.

Spinal Cord Part of the nervous system, contained inside the bony spine and extending from the base of the skull to the lower back.

Spleen Large organ, consisting mainly of lymphocytes (types of white blood cells). It is in the top left-hand side of the abdomen close to the stomach.

Splenectomy Removal of the spleen.

Staging Finding the true extent of disease. This is done in many ways, including surgery and radiology.

Sterility Inability to produce children or freedom from infection.

Stomatitis Inflammation of the mucosa (lining) in the mouth.

Subcutaneous Under the skin.

Suppository Form of medication that is inserted into the rectum.

Thrombocytopenia Below-normal levels of platelets in the blood.

Thorax Chest.

Titration Accurate adjustment (e.g., of a drug dose upwards or downwards).

Ultrasound Sound waves that produce echoes for diagnosis. They are too high-pitched to be heard.

Ureter Tube that carries urine from a kidney to the bladder.

Urinary Tract System for producing, transporting, storing, and excreting urine. The kidneys, ureter, bladder, and urethra (the tube from the bladder to the outside) make up the urinary tract.

Urticaria Hives.

Vaccination Immunization—injections of changed micro-organisms or extracts of them to prevent infection.

Varicella Chicken pox.

Vertebrae Bones making up the spine.

Vesicles Blisters.

VMA/HVA Vanillylmandelic acid and homovanillic acid—products of neuroblastoma cells that are excreted in the urine in large amounts.

White Blood Cells Colorless collection of granulocytes, lymphocytes, and monocytes.

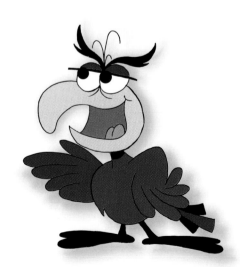

INDEX